Lifescaping Practices in School Communities

Lifescaping Practices in School Communities is a guide for school administrators and helping professionals (school counselors, school psychologists, school social workers, and other stakeholders) looking to promote relational wellness and student success in their school. This informative new resource will introduce readers to an ecological approach by using action research and appreciative inquiry to guide and engage school-wide change. Also offered are first-hand models of conceptual lifescaping projects using action research and appreciative inquiry by first-time practitioners from different school communities.

Rolla E. Lewis, EdD, NCC, is professor emeritus in Educational Psychology at California State University, East Bay (CSUEB). His current research and scholarly interests include public education advocacy, school counseling program development, mentoring participatory leaders, and sharing action research practices using the participatory inquiry process as lifescaping in schools. Dr. Lewis has published numerous chapters, articles, and poems in books, peer-reviewed journals, and other professional publications. He is the recipient of the Oregon Counseling Association's Leona Tyler Award for outstanding contributions to professional counseling.

Peg Winkelman, PhD, is professor and chair in the Department of Educational Leadership at California State University, East Bay (CSUEB). She has also taught in schools of education at the University of California, Berkeley, Mills College, and Saint Mary's College of California. She is past president of the California Association of Professors of Educational Administration. Her publications focus on her commitment to collaborative inquiry and scholar-practitioner leadership for social justice.

"Our goal as educators is to promote ALL children's core gifts. *Lifescaping Practices in School Communities* inspires practitioners to transcend mired systems that reify the status quo in our schools and provides a road map through language and action that harnesses the strengths and voices of our wonderfully diverse communities. As we move from polarization to inclusion, this publication encourages us to move toward a common vision through inclusive practices."

Rose Borunda, EdD, professor, California State
University, Sacramento

"Lewis and Winkelman escape the narrow vision of education that has held schools in its grip recently. Instead, they invite educators and help professionals to soar. Their concept of lifescaping is a big enough vision to inspire education, rather than mere schooling, and becoming somebody distinctive, rather than just fitting in. Their contributors have, moreover, practical suggestions about how to get there, including the use of appreciative inquiry and participatory action research."

John Winslade, PhD, professor, California
State University, San Bernardino

"This book addresses a missing piece in calls for closing achievement gaps. The authors examine student support through a lens of student wellness and an ecological approach to program development, bringing fresh air to discussions of what works. Highlighting action research and appreciative inquiry points the way towards continuous improvement in serving the academic, personal/social, and career development needs of youth. Packed with useful resources and good sense, this volume should become a staple in counselor education and student support programs."

Lonnie L. Rowell, PhD, associate professor, School of Leadership
and Education Sciences, University of San Diego; lead editor,
International Handbook of Action Research

"This scholarly book provides a state-of-the-art, and much needed, contribution to a wide range of school communities: administrators, practitioners, and graduate trainees. The expertly written text successfully infuses theoretical, clinical, and empirical findings into a coherent, well-structured mosaic. It is my belief that this comprehensive work greatly enhances our knowledge of action and participatory research and, therefore, should make a welcome addition to school administration and counseling libraries."

Hanoch Livneh, PhD, LPC, professor emeritus, Counselor
Education, Portland State University Fellow;
American Psychological Association

Lifescaping Practices in School Communities

Implementing Action Research and Appreciative Inquiry

Rolla E. Lewis
and Peg Winkelman

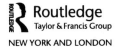

Routledge
Taylor & Francis Group

NEW YORK AND LONDON

First published 2017
by Routledge
711 Third Avenue, New York, NY 10017

and by Routledge
2 Park Square, Milton Park, Abingdon, Oxon, OX14 4RN

*Routledge is an imprint of the Taylor & Francis Group,
an informa business*

Library of Congress Cataloging in Publication Data
A catalog record for this book has been requested

ISBN: 978-1-138-20947-3 (hbk)
ISBN: 978-1-138-20948-0 (pbk)
ISBN: 978-1-315-45713-0 (ebk)

Typeset in Sabon
by Florence Production Limited, Stoodleigh, Devon, UK

Contents

Illustrations

Figures

Tables

Change Activities
Facilitating Action and Movement

Contributors

Lisa Davies, EdD, is currently the Director of Secondary Academics in an urban school district in the San Francisco Bay Area. She holds a Bachelor of Science and Master of Arts degree in Education from San Francisco State University and earned a Doctorate in Educational Leadership from California State University, East Bay. Dr. Davies is dedicated to ensuring that all students have equitable access to rigorous learning opportunities in an effort to make certain they are prepared to be competitive and make a positive difference in our society.

Molly Griffin is a school counselor at Centerville Junior High School in Fremont, CA. Molly is a graduate of California State University, East Bay in 2011, with a Master's degree in Counseling with an emphasis on School Counseling and Marriage and Family Therapy. Molly's current focus is assisting in developing a Multi-Tiered System of Support (MTSS) framework at Centerville to support the academic learning and social/emotional support of all students.

Lisa Maibaum, MS, NSCP, graduated from California State University, East Bay in 2010, with a Master's in Counseling and a PPS Credential in School Psychology. She currently works as a school psychologist in Marin County. She is also a Licensed Educational Psychologist and Licensed Marriage and Family Therapist Intern. Lisa holds an Education Specialist Credential and has taught adolescents in a day treatment setting. Her scholarly interests include equity and disproportionality, adolescent development, social–emotional well-being, and treating students with mental health concerns in schools.

Kathryn (Katie) Messina is a Counselor/Instructor at Chabot College. She earned her Master's degree in Counseling/Pupil Personnel Services Credential from California State University, East Bay (CSUEB) in 2014, Master's degree in Education/Teaching Credential from Stanford University in 2006, and Bachelor's degree in Sociology from University of California, Los Angeles (UCLA) in 2003. She has over ten years' experience as a public school educator working with diverse middle school, high school, and college student populations.

Foreword

Kenneth J. Gergen
The Taos Institute

Like all major institutions, schools emerge from within the currents of cultural process, and they inevitably reflect the values and assumptions of these surrounds. Just as many institutions of government and commerce, schools thus serve as concrete representations of these assumptions and values. Such institutions are like stakes in the ground, flags unfurled, proclaiming themselves to be enduring symbols of a valued way of life. Yet, while schools are established to maintain a given way of life, the way of life continues to change. In spite of the solid structures, the culture moves on. And especially within recent decades, the magnitude of these changes is breathtaking. Almost half the world's population is now connected by internet, with over 140 million email messages a second now circling the globe. Over a billion migrants move across borders and into new cultures. Everywhere there are new ideas, inspirations, transformations, and hybrids in motion. In contrast, schools are largely conservative institutions. They are lodged in a discourse of "basics," "foundations," "universals," "traditions," and the like. They are little given to absorbing the currents of change.

We thus find ourselves in a condition in which our educational practices are increasingly less reflective of the cultural conditions. Or, one might say, our educational institutions are becoming increasingly irrelevant. This rapidly emerging dislocation is no surprise to teachers, students, and administrators. Many educators are indeed on the forefront in demanding change. There is, of course, the continuing problem of squeezing funds from the public coffers to sustain our educational institutions, much less improve them. And there are problems of equalizing educational opportunities across lines of race, social class, and ethnicity. But one of the central if not pivotal shortcomings lies within the walls of the school building, where students find little of interest or meaning in their classrooms, and teachers are frustrated with sullen, uninterested, and unruly students. Both students and teachers also labor under the pervasive threat of "being measured." Drop-out rates continue unabated, and home schooling becomes an increasingly attractive alternative. There is little vitality in these cultures of learning.

It is in this context that I find myself impressed, illuminated, and inspired by the present offering. Here Rolla Lewis, Peg Winkelman and their associates confront the emerging condition with creative daring. Rather than writing yet another critique of what's wrong, they offer a virtual road map to an exciting future. They offer teachers, school counselors, and administrators a rationale for new forms of action, a new range of challenging practices, and useful applications of their orientation in action. There is no easy way to summarize this extensive work; the scholarly scope is enormous, the nuances numerous, and the associated ideas expansive. However, I would like to highlight three major lines of development that had me singing lustily alongside the authors and their associates:

From Autonomy to Collaboration. Traditional institutions of education are based on the longstanding Western vision of individual rationality. Emerging from Greek philosophy, buttressed by Christianity, and elaborated by modernist thinkers from Descartes to contemporary cognitivists, society is essentially viewed as a collection of rational and self-directed individuals. Within education this view is reflected not only in the focus on filling and testing individual minds, but as well in the hierarchical structure of the educational system. The result in the educational sphere is pervasive oppression and alienation. Pointing to deep deficiencies in this tradition, Lewis and Winkelman bring into view the enormous potentials inhering in collaborative process. With the realization that our conceptions of the world and the values we place on our actions emerge from processes of relationship, they see appreciative and collaborative practices as a cornerstone for vitalizing communities of learning. Participatory inquiry serves as a key practice for transformation.

Value Restoration. The dominant view of knowledge within the educational sphere places an emphasis on reason and evidence. Values, on this account, are personal and subjective. The outcome of this view is that issues of value, desire, or morality are either hidden within the curriculum, or entirely eliminated from discussion. Translated into student terms, there is little in the curriculum that one "cares about." Classes proceed without passion. Here Lewis and Winkelman again step into the breach. In their view, matters of value should play a central role in developing communities of learning. As their discussion of appreciative practices makes clear, it is when collaborative activities center on that which we value, learning is a natural outcome. We wish to learn, because it is the means of realizing our hopes for a better world. In the present volume, the point is effectively made through discussions of environmental sustainability and social justice. When such values are placed in the forefront, education is energized.

Future Making. Educational systems are largely premised on a vision of knowledge as a preparatory resource. That is, we assume that knowledge makers provide sound reflections of the world as it is, and that by mastering these reflections, students will be equipped to make rationally adaptive decisions in later life. While this assumption is open to debate on many counts, it also carries a strongly conserving force. In brief, it suggests that without mastering existing knowledge, one is ill equipped to take action. One is not invited to dream, to plan, or to initiate change, but to wait until the "mind has been filled." Lewis and Winkelman are well aware of the enervating effect of these pervasive assumptions, and thus offer a counter proposal: engage the learning community in future making! Draw from the wellsprings of value, and concomitant search for meaningful knowledge, they reason, and set out to affect the order of things. Here the authors make use of the inviting metaphor of lifescaping, a way of approaching the future as an engaged participant in creating a better world.

Of course, I would like to think that my writings have added energy to the efforts of these authors. And while they suggest as much, I believe I have provided little more than an insignia. Lewis, Winkelman, and their associates drew the power for this volume from their own collaborative, passionate, and future forming activities together. Their knowledge and inspiration grows from their immersion in action. My deepest hope is that what they share within this work can ignite a thousand fires.

Acknowledgments

No book is the sole creation of its authors. Although authors are responsible for any errors and omissions, as authors, we are always mindful how we are tied in relational webs to others we have talked to, been taught by, whose work we have read, or stumbled upon in many different ways. The text becomes an expression of what we capture in sharing our lived experience and reflection upon what we have done to construct learning communities that promote learning power and relational well-being. The text becomes a snapshot at a certain moment of time. It is not offering some static truth. The text merely provides a certain evolving perspective.

Schools, universities, and professional organizations can function as villages that foster learning power and well-being. There will be many villagers who go unnamed in any thank you or acknowledgement; in schools, these are the secretaries, the custodians, the aides, and others who offer everyday comfort and support to the children and professionals who enter the school community. We want to thank the unnamed for the comfort and support they have provided to our students and us. Thanks to the Oregon School Counselor Association for the many conversations and continuing support. Thanks to the Oregon Counseling Association for their abundant support, especially when Rolla was president of the Oregon Association for Counselor Education and Supervision.

Those individuals who have been most helpful, we want to recognize our chapter authors for their contributions: Molly Griffin, Lisa Maibaum, Katie Messina, and Lisa Davies stepped forward to offer examples of the evolving participatory inquiry process (PIP) and how their conversations and work impacted what they did in their schools to help kids. We want to thank Greg Jennings for his comments on the first draft of the book. Laurie Huntwork offered kind comments on a very early draft. Thanks to Bradley Porfilio for his early critical review of the text. Special thanks to Hanoch Livneh for his critical review and for mentoring Rolla early in his career in higher education. Thanks to David Capuzzi for pointing us to Routledge and for his help in sharing our work. Thanks to Christopher Teja of Routledge for his encouragement and support. My deep appreciation for their encouragement to career mentors Carol Burden, Joan Avis,

Iris St. John, and Elaina Rose Lovejoy. Kudos to Re'nice Siefer for modeling excellence in school counseling and for being an ally.

The work and encouragement of Kenneth Gergen is woven into the text; when we recognized that Ken's world forming construct resonated with our lifescaping notion, we were thrilled. John Winslade has been a generous influence in the narrative threads in this work.

The professionals-in-training at California State University, East Bay have been inspirational. They are the ones who pressed us to write the book. Mary Champion and Emily Santiago offered their insights to an early draft. Bethany Toy used a later draft to guide her powerful appreciative inquiry and action research in her school. The graduate students who have used this work were all instrumental in helping us to balance grounding our text in a theoretical perspective and offering very practical steps for doing the work.

Lonnie Rowell is a leader in the school counseling action research community. Rolla deeply appreciates his wisdom and insights into using action research as a tool for promoting social justice; his Social Publishers Foundation is a resource and inspiration to all of us. Bonnie Benard showed Rolla how to integrate resilience into his work as a school counselor and counselor educator. When at WestEd, Bonnie's work with Sara Truebridge and Sean Slade offered much hope for promoting better learning futures for all students.

Deep appreciation and thanks to our colleagues at CSUEB: Jack Davis, Oanh Tran, Janet Logan, Bradley Porfilio, Provost Carolyn Nelson, and Dean James Zarillo.

Rolla appreciates the conversations with friends and family that have added to and contributed a certain life perspective. Thanks to Ellen Singer, Ed Vine, Paul and Mari Litsky, Barbara and Denis Schmidt, Glenn and Monet Rubin, Michael and Evelyn Seeger. Rolla's children Alexandra Lewis, Ryan Lewis, and Glenn Semrad have given him different takes on what it means to construct a satisfying life; they instill in him the hope that future generations will lifescape a more just, compassionate, and relational world.

Most of all, Rolla wants to thank his partner, Cornelia Lewis, for being supportive when he disappeared into the study to write and for being compassionate when he came out of the study feeling stuck. Cornelia and her sister, Sibylle Scharer, and her friends, Rachel Bradley and Linda Hennessey, have been his muses.

Introduction

> We live in a world in which religious and political conflict threaten the globe, . . . communities are eroding, longstanding cultural traditions are evaporating, and we struggle with our relationships to our habitat . . . It is time . . . to channel . . . intelligence and ingenuity into creating more flourishing forms of living together.
>
> (Kenneth J. Gergen, 2015)

In the article "From mirroring to world-making: Research as future forming," Ken Gergen (2015) offered the understanding that action research can be a practice designed to explore and create possible futures that are more life-enhancing. By shifting research from merely mirroring what is thought to be into an active effort to create a world that can be, Gergen conceptualized an action-oriented process where research is used by local practitioners to work within communities and organizations to construct the world where they want to live and grow. In Chapter 1, we refer to this process as lifescaping. Lifescaping is action directed toward cultivating learning power and well-being in schools, organizations, and communities. Terms such as "future forming" and "lifescaping" move research away from being a descriptive summary of what and how the world is toward research being a creative and continuous process of becoming and making the world we desire. Lifescaping is about enacting and performing what Wittgenstein (1953) called new forms of life. The shift to using terms such as "future forming" and "lifescaping" is both radical and vital.

The two specific approaches to future forming research discussed in Gergen's article are action research and appreciative inquiry, which are the two practices being shared in this book designed to support education advocates in creating better futures for students in their schools. We knew both action research and appreciative inquiry were powerful tools for fostering creative systemic change, and we wanted to develop a text that might help guide student advocates (administrators, school counselors, school psychologists, school social workers, teachers, parents, students, and other community members) in creating school communities that actively support student well-being and learning power—schools that students, parents, communities, and professionals want.

We were reflecting on our first draft of the book when we read Dr. Gergen's (2015) seminal article. The article opened our eyes and deepened our understanding and appreciation for action research and appreciative inquiry as "future forming" approaches for creating new worlds—different ways of being in school communities. The article also helped us to see that our notion of a "lifescaping" construct aligned with Dr. Gergen's world forming concept. We understood action research as a creative act, and our action-oriented approach focused on describing the process, actions, and results as integral to reflective practitioner practice. Our work is designed to disrupt fixed mindsets where the world is as seen and acted upon as somewhat static, "the way it is"; we invite readers to embrace growth mindsets where the world is understood as being actively formed through an engaged and inclusive inquiry process. The "mindset" construct emerged from Carol Dweck's (2006) research regarding successful learners; students with growth mindsets see their minds as muscles to be exercised and developed, whereas students with fixed mindsets see their brains as limited to what they were born with or the way it is. We see mindsets as emerging in discourse rather than merely contained in individual heads. How do the family, school, and community support growth mindset discourses rather than promote fixed mindset discourses. How do professionals in schools promote a growth mindset discourse where all students are viewed as learners, rather than as some being smart and others dumb? Expanded into discourse, Dweck's growth mindset notion permeates our work, and as we see it, Gergen's future forming construct is about cultivating relational growth mindsets within individuals, groups, and institutions.

Reading Dr. Gergen's article was a discovery and affirmation, as if someone had gifted us with a term that was just beyond the tip of our tongues but not in our lexicon, like the early European explorers who found what they thought was a "new world" but did not have the word "discovery" in their lexicon (Wootton, 2015). We realized that our work was about world forming in schools, and that future forming and lifescaping were related terms concerned with helping groups and communities create the world they want to live in. The term shook us to our core. Every student advocate (administrator, helping professional, teacher, parent, student, and community member) who cares about schools as learning communities dreams of creating better futures for students. Our dream is that this archetypal educator dream includes ALL kids as active agents in their own learning communities where they are supported in living into their greatest potential as citizens and workers. Furthermore, our dream is for school communities to recognize them as existing in social and biological ecologies that we are part of, not separate from the world around us—we as humans are part of the social ecologies and life ecologies where we work and dwell. As the Union of Concerned Scientists says, we can no longer deny the human impact of global warming (Global Warming Science, n.d.). Braidotti (2013) describes how we all exist within a vital geo-centrism that defines life as a constant flow. We also exist in an era being defined as the "anthropocene age" that defines humans as a geological force capable of affecting all life on this planet. Humans are changing the climate. Life is surging. Anthropologists such as Tim Ingold (2011) have looped back to exploring what it means to be alive; we are all enmeshed in living; no single thread can capture the complex weave that is life. Theologians such as Cupitt (1999, 2003) point out that in the West life is the sacred object. We resonate with the belief that each student's life should be revered and that all students should be recognized as resources and participants in a living learning community, not a Kafkaesque bureaucratic maze designed and defined by others who have no connection to or deep knowledge of the community where the students attend school.

We humans are active agents of planetary change, but are very much part of the living earth we are changing and the communities where we dwell. Such a topic as the ecological destruction of Earth is well-beyond the scope of this text, but even in that, our response to the massive global challenges is to explore what we can do in local school communities to foster the relational bond that connects, that fosters local knowledge and practices, and provides practical tools that might help us take action toward forming positive futures in the places where we work with kids and live our lives. Our work is local and framed always in terms of what will work and what can be adapted for use in differing but specific communities consisting of diverse people living in unique bio-ecosystems and human microsystems. We are not offering some universal plan; only tools for taking action and a perspective that might help guide future forming and lifescaping actions. Our work takes place in local and specific schools in Northern California that range from communities with very few resources to communities that have abundant resources, from urban to suburban to rural communities, from communities with shifting demographics composed of groups including African-American, Latino, Asian, Middle Eastern-American, Native-American, European-American to less diverse communities. We are from California where there is no longer a majority racial or ethnic population, but there are "haves" and "have-nots" in every community. Each community has its own challenges, but clearly with the opportunity gap, digital gap, income gap, education gap, achievement gap, etc., some communities need more support and resources than others in order to help kids reach their greatest potential as citizens and human beings.

The relationship and connection to ecosystems can be emotional and personal (Mehl-Madrona, 2005, 2010; Milton, 2002). Ecosystems connect to the biological and to social systems. For instance, Rolla remembers the influence of growing up as a kid in elementary school, remembers catching blue belly and horned lizards along the Rio San Gabriel; and remembers reading John Muir (1894/1961) and Aldo Leopold (1949) in high school and as an undergraduate as the first member of his family to go to college. In high school, Rolla also worked as a delivery boy for Edward Gallardo, a first-generation Mexican-American florist who loved to take Rolla to the commercial flower market in downtown Los Angeles and parts of the city where Spanish was the first language. Connection to where he lived and traveled has always had a profound impact upon how Rolla views his relationship and responsibility toward the environment to which we belong. When John Muir (1894/1961) talked about climbing a Douglas Spruce during a Sierra Nevada storm and "travel[ing] the milky way together" with the tree, he opened Rolla up to a certain feeling toward trees (p. 196). Rolla's appreciation and understanding for those words deepened experientially when he climbed a valley oak during a rainstorm, swaying back and forth in the limbs, learning that empathy grows from active and engaged relationships. Aldo Leopold (1949) moved Rolla toward a deeper appreciation of ecological responsibility and ethics stating, "When we see land as a community to which we belong ... is the basic concept of ecology, but that land is to be loved and respected is an extension of ethics" (p. viii). Ethics will be discussed more in this text, but for now it is important to understand that ethics are connected to obligations, responsibility, and actions—what we do. This definition of ethics must be evoked among the adults who support students and should be embedded in our work for and with students so that they experience the positive power of ethical action and community.

Peg grew up with a love for learning in and outside the classroom; yet a "nagging" sense of social responsibility developed with each year she spent in California public schools. From kindergarten through her completion of a Ph.D. program at the University of California, Berkeley, Peg found that she consistently held a privileged position, possessing social and cultural capital that was not shared by all her classmates in K-12 schools, undergraduate or graduate programs. When a kindergarten teacher thought "Peggy" might not be ready for first grade because she couldn't use scissors, Peggy's college-educated mother requested a conference, questioning the relevance of "cutting" to academic pursuits such as reading, solving mathematical problems, or providing a scientific hypothesis (all of which her mother insisted Peggy was capable of doing at age five). Though her family moved frequently, Peggy never spent more than a day in the lowest reading group. When the fourth grade science curriculum seemed weak, her mother started an after-school science club. When Peggy started high school, she was placed in a Chemistry course for juniors and seniors. Again her mother was able to support Peggy and her timid lab partner through all the college prep work. With homework support and her parents' knowledge of the college application process, it was not surprising that she was accepted to her first choice college. Throughout her undergraduate and graduate years, Peg recognized that she had been born into an advantaged social, economic, and educational position. As she tutored students from impoverished neighborhoods and schools she found her passion for serving students. Peg's lived experience compelled her to examine inequities in schools and connect with student advocates to create greater educational opportunity for under-served students and marginalized communities. Peg and Rolla connected through a common commitment to lifescaping and future forming practices.

The text we are offering is about providing graduate students, professionals-in-training, practicing school administrators, teachers, counselors, school psychologists, social workers, students, and community members, all of whom are working on behalf of students, tools for engaging in future forming practices that support students' well-being and learning power. In other words, what we offer is conceptual but, more importantly, our hope is that the practical tools presented create pragmatic relational changes that form better futures for all students and the communities where they dwell. We address our readers as advocates, for if one chooses to read a book with "lifescaping" in the title, we feel it is safe to assume that the reader is a student advocate.

Why write this book? For each of us, neither of us had a text we could pull off the shelf that would meet our needs in teaching graduate students and practicing professionals how to promote transformative change in schools. We had a host of articles and texts that captured this or that part of what we were trying to say, but there was no core text that captured the future forming and lifescaping relational practices being presented in this text. Rolla's school psychology students will have to forgive his bias but at heart he is a school counselor, and a part of what is written is about creating pathways for constructing comprehensive school counseling programs that serve all youth by promoting learning power and well-being. The book actually emerged from pressure by professionals-in-training who asked Rolla to put what he was saying into one source they could follow in a way that helped them achieve effective results without having to read so many different assigned resources. It was the work of our graduate students that brought us into collaboration on this publication. At the 2013 American Educational Research Association (AERA) Conference doctoral students in the Educational Leadership for Social Justice program presented their participatory action research side-by-side with MS in Counseling students, and Peg got a glimpse of the connections between her work in Educational Leadership and the expertise of Rolla Lewis in Educational Psychology. We hope the book serves to guide positive and life-enhancing systems change in schools. We offer this approach with a humble reverence for those whose shoulders we stand upon as authors.

We hope this text will provide our readers, student advocates, the tools necessary to conduct action research and appreciative inquiry as ongoing lifescaping practices that build relationships that promote well-being and learning power in local school communities. The dialogical nature of the text means that in our professional relationships there will be conversations and a continuous inquiry into what is seen, what is heard, and the impact of the actions we take with others.

This text is divided into three parts. Part one offers a conceptual overview, grounding readers in the roots of and ideas guiding our work. It offers both a personal and professional perspective about the work. Part I has five chapters. Chapter 1 offers a philosophical overview of the practice and introduces the term "lifescaping" as action taken to promote the learning power and well-being of all, including students, staff, faculty, administrators, helping professionals, and community members. Chapter 2 expands on Chapter 1 by providing the context of schools as relational ecosystems and defining the construct of learning power. Chapter 3 illuminates the importance of utilizing (recognizing and interrogating) school narratives to inform inquiry and positive action. What are the stories kids or adults share about your school? How are professionals taking steps to create more playful and nurturing learning experiences at your school? Chapter 4 introduces the participatory inquiry process (PIP), a lifescaping action research process developed to help advocates working with students, parents, teachers, administrators, and other stakeholders take action and document the action steps they take in their school. Chapter 5 introduces a four-phase relational (4-R) appreciative inquiry process, a lifescaping practice designed to build on the existing positive core in the school where you work. The appreciative process creates the relational context (the how) for a participatory inquiry focused on better serving students (the what).

Part II is a sequential description where each chapter describes each phase of both PIP and the 4-R appreciative inquiry (AI) process. Chapter 6 details both PIP Phase 1: Initiating Conversations and Identifying Challenges, and AI Phase 1: Relational Connection. Chapter 7 presents both PIP Phase 2: Engaged Inquiry, and AI Phase 2: Relational Dialogue. Chapter 8 portrays both PIP Phase 3: Collaborative Action, and AI Phase 3: Relational Action. Chapter 9 describes both PIP Phase 4: Community Assessment and Reflection, and AI Phase 4: Relational Assessment and Reflection.

Part III of the book consists of chapters by actual graduate students, professionals-in-training who used PIP to guide their work in the schools during their graduate degree programs. The work is written by beginning professionals and is presented in a manner that maintains their voice, their wonderings, and their beginning steps as practitioners using the tools described in this text. Maintaining the beginning professional voice was vital and both co-authors positioned and restrained ourselves to do anything other than have the authors align their work with the action research participatory inquiry process being presented in this text.

The references and resources that inform and guide this work are extensive. We have tried to provide a comprehensive list that includes websites and references to the work we have used and the shoulders we stand upon in writing this work. If you sense that we have failed to recognize any names or resources, please let us know. The Appendices are oriented to moving the practice along and present tools that will help practitioners during each phase of either PIP or the AI process.

We wish you success and joy in your future forming and lifescaping efforts.

Part I

Action Research as a Participatory Inquiry Process and an Appreciative Inquiry Process

Continuous Dialogues and Actions in School Communities

1 Eco-Relational Lifescaping in Schools

The values that have allowed Western capitalism to thrive now threaten its collapse: commitment to parts, divisions, individualism, competition, utility, efficiency, simplicity, choice, consumption, busyness, excess, growth, and speed—above all, speed. And the values this regime has repressed now need to be cultivated: commitment to the whole, relationships, community cooperation, generosity, patience, subtlety, deliberation, analysis, complexity, uncertainty, leisure, and reflection—above all reflection.

(Mark C. Taylor, 2014, p. 343)

The analogy, then, is not between society and organism as entities, but between social *life* and organic *life* understood as processes.

(Tim Ingold, 2011, p. 234; emphasis in original)

Feeling at home in life is for me one of the many purposes in living . . . To feel at home in life requires both the willpower and the desire to participate in it actively.

(Arne Naess, 2002, p. 2)

As noted in the introduction, this book is designed as a guide for student advocates (school counselors, school psychologists, school social workers, school administrators, teachers, parents, students, and other community members) interested in promoting student and school community strengths via future forming and lifescaping actions directed toward cultivating learning power and well-being in schools, organizations, and communities. Lifescaping and future forming move research away from being a descriptive summary or trying to be a mirror of reality toward action research becoming an engaged creative and continuous process directed toward making schools, organizations, and communities better places for living and learning. The content in this text orients readers to strengths-based eco-relational change practices to be implemented in school communities. Strengths-based practices in the schools is an approach that builds on strengths rather than attempting merely to minimize deficits and problems (e.g., Galassi & Akos, 2007). Eco-relational change is a term that merges ecological counseling (Conyne & Cook, 2004) with the relational insights being forwarded in social constructionist psychology and deep ecology philosophy (e.g., Gergen, 2009; Naess, 2002; Spretnak, 2011). Eco-relational change is concerned with the complex ecologies where we exist and enhancing the relationships in those ecologies that promote connection, belongingness, integrity, compassion, and human potential.

The action research participatory inquiry process (PIP) and the appreciative inquiry (AI) process described in this text are practices for student advocates who want to engage in future forming and lifescaping change at their school. The practices in this book draw upon core sources, but should be viewed like jazz, where there are relational and contextual variations to the genre, such as East Coast, West Coast, French, Gypsy, Latin, and numerous other jazz styles. Cornel West describes jazz "not so much as a term for a musical art form but for a mode of being in the world, an improvisational mode of protean, fluid and flexible disposition toward reality suspicious of 'either/or' viewpoints" (1993, p. 150). The strengths-based practices described here are a form of jazz that is relational, collaborative, and dialogical; what we refer to as eco-relational. The eco-relational perspective described in this text is an integration of theories rooted in the strengths-based perspective described by Galassi and Akos (2007), the ecological perspective developed by Bronfenbrenner (1979), Conyne and Cook (2004), and Naess (2002), the learning and development theory offered by Vygotsky and his adherents (1978, 1986; Holzman, 1997; Newman & Holzman, 1993, 1996; van der Veer & Valsiner, 1994), and the social constructionist and relational work exemplified by Gergen (2006, 2009). Each has framed their approach to relationships and counseling ways that allow for creative play and new practices while maintaining an essential social constructionist, strengths-based, and ecological core that draws on the vitality of relational integrity. The eco-relational approach described in the text is personal, relational, dialogical, and storied; the text uses the jazz metaphor to heighten listening and improvisation as vital to our work; the text also uses a gardening metaphor to boost the notion of creatively working with what is, planting what will grow in the living context, and continuously adapting, changing, weeding, and watering over time to lifescape the world you desire. Jazz and gardening are similar in that they improvise to what is offered up or presented; both constantly adjust to the context and circumstances to make the best choice in the moment with the materials at hand, only jazz actions pass in that moment the music is played while the results of gardening actions might not be realized for some time after the season has passed or moved beyond planting again.

We as authors are not separate from the ecological systems we describe; we are participants who have had to adapt, adjust, and survive in our own unique ways in the life-generating systems where we exist. The style described in this text draws upon Greg Jennings' (2012) notion of orienting student advocates to the importance of having "professional mojo" or self-assuredness, skilled responsiveness in uncertain situations where they find themselves, and having the personal power to tap what Werner and Smith (1992) storied over forty years as human resilience that enables people to spring back from setbacks and other obstacles, as well as assert themselves positively and creatively in the systems and relationships where they live out their careers and lives. Our job as student advocates in the schools is to foster what Ann Masten calls the ordinary magic of developmental resilience by creating structures that support students and assessing how well what we are doing works to promote their success. The eco-relational approach draws upon educational researcher Lisa Delpit's tenets to recognize and use experiences from a child's world to connect what they already know to school knowledge and create a sense of caring community in the service of academic achievement (Delpit, 2006). PIP and AI align with what is referred to in educational leadership research as collaborative inquiry (Copland, 2003; Herman & Gribbons, 2001; Huffman & Kalnin, 2003; Storms & Gordon, 2005; Winkelman, 2012). Educational administrators benefit from a counseling perspective as they develop their leadership capacity in what Fullan (2001) describes as "relationship building."

Strengths-based eco-relational counseling is a certain way of thinking and relating in the world as a student advocate. The eco-relational approach embraces a deep understanding that humans must learn to see themselves as citizens in a living community ecosphere, just as they are challenged to be open-minded and contributing citizens in their local communities. Indigenous and First Nations cultures have recognized the person and land connection for eons, and Native-American scholars have asserted the need to integrate Indigenous or First Nations knowledges and wisdom into the wider community via environmental education and counseling practice to promote greater connectedness between people and the land where they dwell (e.g., Kapyrka & Dockstator, 2012; Mehl-Madrona, 2005, 2007, 2010). Indeed, similar to what this text offers, relationality is at the heart of what it means to be Indigenous and to the Indigenous research methodology (Wilson, 2008). For First Nations people, everything emerges from relationships. The same holds for the eco-relational approach, which calls for relational understanding and, we believe, what Claxton (1997) calls "poetic sensibility." At the school and community level, eco-relational counseling is concerned with relationships, between, among, and where relationships are located historically; eco-relational counseling in the schools is also concerned with exploring the positive core and bringing out the best possibilities for promoting the learning power and well-being of all members of the school community.

The practices in the book are designed to support student advocates in developing an eco-relational understanding, forms of engagement, and the capacity to move with members of their school community to create a greater sense of well-being and learning power for everyone. The only genuine way to learn the approach is active engagement in the relationships and ecosystems where people live and work. In fact, everything said and suggested in this text has to be adjusted to the local and specific context where the student advocate finds him or herself. The Bibliography is meant to invite advocates to take a deeper look at what is presented and to be able to explore and use the rich sources that are cited. In this book, professionals we have taught in our work as professors have developed the examples from their practice in the schools in their local communities.

It is important to note that this book is not for armchair reading. The book is an action-oriented guide for iterative relational reflection that invites an ongoing cycle of inquiry in the schools. The strengths-based eco-relational text orients readers to lifescaping practices that benefit and engage the school community. The target audience is anyone committed to better serving students including (but not limited to) school administrators, teacher leaders, activity directors, school counselors, school psychologists, school social workers, students, and community members. In this text we will generally refer to our readers as student advocates. Anyone engaged in this pursuit is, by definition, a student advocate for helping all students live up to their life potential and for helping school communities become vibrant places that foster and enhance life's possibilities.

The text is guided by Gergen's (2015) notion of action research and appreciative inquiry as future forming practices or what we call lifescaping practices; future forming and lifescaping turn research into an active and ongoing process for collaboratively creating more life-affirming futures in the schools. In some ways, the future never arrives because we are always in process, moving, adapting, and changing, and in lifescaping there is also always something more to do to keep nurturing what we have planted and in keeping the weeds out of the garden. Still, we can choose to engage in local and specific actions designed to create and inform greater possibilities for all youth. The action research and the appreciative inquiry methods shared in this text are tools for what we refer to as lifescaping or the engaged process of taking action to create a better world with others at your school, one that promotes the well-being and learning power of students and those working in your learning community.

Schools as Learning Communities

Our definition of learning community extends beyond the current practice of professional learning communities and moves toward encouraging schools to become communities of practice. The professional learning community (PLC) described in educational leadership literature typically focuses only on collaboration among teachers (Darling-Hammond, Chung, Andree, Richardson, & Orphanos, 2009; DuFour, 2006; Louis, 1994). Often school counselors, school psychologists, school social workers, parents, other community members, and students themselves are only invited to discuss the learning of individual students. Studies consistently link professional collaboration to increased student achievement (Louis & Marks, 1998; Goddard et al., 2007; Bryk et al., 2010; Odden & Archibald, 2009). We propose that expanding opportunities for dialogue and collaboration as well as the inquiry "data" utilized in collaboration with key participants will further students' learning power and civic engagement in their school as a community of practice. In this book we encourage readers to consider a school community collaboration and inquiry inclusive of all who are concerned with the relational wellness and learning power of students and to place the lived experiences of students at the center of all work.

Schools are learning communities where we humans, facing a vast and endless cosmos and a world filled with myriad uncertainties, create space where respectful relationships can be fostered and opportunities that promote the relational wellness and learning power of students can be established as core guiding principles. This book is about seeing, hearing, and speaking out about the importance of positive relationships, promoting relational wellness, and unleashing students' learning power.

The notion of learning power was coined by Claxton (1999), and has evolved into an approach for transforming how teaching and learning are approached in schools (Claxton, 2002; Claxton et al., 2011; Claxton & Lucas, 2015). As used in this text, the learning power construct builds on Claxton and on Dweck (2006) to include Vygotsky's (Holzman, 1997) notion that learning is fostered and development is enhanced by how we relate to each other, as humans living life, as students, and as teachers. Learning power is not passive; learning power is an active belief and process focused on vital engagement and doing things that are meaningful to learners while fostering their academic (head), personal/social (heart), and work/career (hands) development (Hatch & Lewis, 2011). Supported by a wise teacher or guide, learning power grows with a sense of competence in actively engaging in self-determined tasks alone or with others. Learning power does not fall into the dualistic trap of pitting high-status abstract knowledge against low-status practical knowledge (Bowers, 2001, 2003). Science and Math are important and so are Shop, Art, Music and other forms of learning for many different students. What is framed as high-status and low-status knowledge are fundamental and both abstract and practical knowledge are needed when integrating head, heart, and hand (3-H) education with the relational connections between and among people within the life-systems where they develop and play (Gandhi, 1953; Goleman et al., 2012; Hatch & Lewis, 2011; Spretnak, 2011; Williams & Brown, 2012). One of the many tragedies in current educational policy in the United States is the obsession with putting going to college for everyone at the expense of and utter failure to include and enhance pathways for students to find significant internships, trades, and other opportunities for meaningful development in their own preferred career and life interests. The discourse about what constitutes meaningful learning must be expanded to include all forms of learning, such as the industrial arts, culinary arts, etc.

Lifescaping

We recognize that each of us is part of a multi-cultural flow that is informed by the chronological (time) and ecological (both biological and social) context where we grow up and live. We are contextualized in multiple ecosystems (Neufeldt & Nelson, 2004). Popular culture, school, social relationships, family, and the space where we live and play shape who we become and how we view the world. This active process to bring about the world we envision is lifescaping, a verb describing the creative and engaged actions planned or taken to shape the world emerging from our own and our communities' unique moment-to-moment perspectives. Lifescaping is world forming in action; like gardeners landscaping, we can take an active role in creatively shaping the world in the social and biological ecosystems where we live. Lifescaping involves dialogical relationships that shape perspectives, understanding, and actions taken toward a desired end. Lifescaping is creating and enacting what the philosopher Ludwig Wittgenstein (1953) called a "new form of life" brought about by the activity of speaking language. We seek allies and communities that will talk to us about and support our active lifescaping and the lifescape we see.

"Lifescaping" draws upon landscape, which is about shaping the land. "Scape" comes from Old English *sceppan* or *skyppan*, meaning "to shape" (Olwig, 2008, cited in Ingold, 2011, p. 126). Lifescaping draws upon landscaping, which is active and engaged, even when defining trails in wilderness areas. Like the diverse forms of landscaping, lifescaping involves understanding culture, environment, and the selection of the right plantings. Lifescape draws upon landscape in a similar manner, one that involves design and perspective, as well as diverse materials. Attempting to impose learning lifescapes that work in one community upon another community will not necessarily thrive; successful lifescaping takes into account the local ecological community and context. Conceptually, lifescape and lifescaping draw upon Husserl's (1936) *Lebenswelt* (lifeworld), but lifescaping builds upon Ingold's (2011) exploration of von UexKull's concept of *Umwelt* (lifespace/environment). Further, the lifescaping and lifescape constructs are informed by Ingold's (2011) notions of entanglement and meshwork, which pose we are all living in entangled social and biological meshworks.

Lifescaping is the act of creatively moving, living, and shaping the discourse and community environment by people. Lifescaping is the changing and adapting perspective that emerges from participation in reflective thought, engaged conversations, and the elegance of actions. Lifescaping can shift fluidly moment-to-moment in relationships over time, during conversations, and in the course of taking action. Yet, our lifescaping takes place in the moment; our lifescape perspective emerges as we experience location and time in our own unique ways within communities of practice where we dwell, work, and, most importantly, prepare to act. Exploring lifescapes involves reflecting upon personal and collective perspectives that inform our seeing and acting along the many pathways we might pursue. In lifescaping we open our lives in our families, at work, at school, and in our communities, as well as with the natural world to different ways of being with ourselves and relating to others. The point in sharing this is that as we bump around our world traveling in lifescapes and lifescaping where we dwell, we are informed by this specific relationship, these unique connections, that particular text; we are influenced by this lecture, television show, movie, play, teacher, mentor, community, etc. We bump around and learn formally and informally, lifescaping our everyday lives as best we can.

Rebecca Solnit (2014) makes this connection: "Everyone is influenced by those things that precede formal education, that come out of the blue and out of everyday life" (p. 73). In our everyday life and our moment-to-moment lifescaping, we create our relational world; we cultivate relationships, play, reflect on ideas, and take actions to construct satisfying lives for ourselves and those we love. Native-American psychiatrist Lewis Mehl-Madrona puts it this way, "There is no individual apart from the milieu in which the individual dwells. This milieu includes the geological world as well as the human world. The indigenous healers . . . would add that it also includes the spirit world" (2005, p. 101). Mehl-Madrona is on to something when we take into account the evolving definition offered by Sheldrake (2014) who says, " 'spirituality' stands for lifestyles and practices that, explicitly or implicitly, portray a vision of human existence and of how our human spirits may achieve their fullest potential" (p. 1). Alexander (2008) asserts that "psychosocial integration is an essential part of human well-being" that must be enhanced if we are going to confront the sense of dislocation and spiritual poverty that lead to addiction and other forms of social disease (p. 85). In *Refiguring the spiritual*, Taylor (2012) shows how contemporary artists, such as Beuys, Barney, Turrell, and Goldsworthy, are renewing ancient spiritual traditions and confronting our current "crisis of vision" (p. 190). Taylor goes on to assert, "vision involves nothing less than the creation of the world . . . *to see differently is to be different*" (italics in original, p. 191). Lifescaping is about seeing the world differently and changing the discourse in the schools where we find ourselves. In lifescaping our everyday practices point toward actively living out ways to live into our own fullest potential while creating space with others in our lives and communities to live into their fullest potential.

We join with others to lifescape new forms of family, school, and community life. Lifescaping efforts are local, but informed by the global.

Lifescaping draws upon Dweck's (2006) growth mindset where intelligence and capability are viewed as muscles, in contrast to the fixed mindset that views intelligence as limited to the brains given at birth. We view mindset as nurtured and fostered in discourse, not as mere possessions of individuals. The growth mindset encourages effort and grit, whereas the fixed mindset can lead to resignation and avoidance. The growth mindset is nurtured in relationships; an individual does not cultivate and develop a growth mindset in isolation. This is a very important point because if mindsets are understood as merely being something that is taught or poured into students, the conversation can quickly degrade into a deficit discourse where students "do not have enough of this or that mindset." Mindsets are fostered and nurtured in conversations in departments, schools, families, and communities. The growth mindset emerges in discourses that support it, and not as an object put into the heads of kids. As well meaning as they are, the ASCA (2014) Mindset Standards fall prey to teaching students "standard" mindsets. Mindsets are taught or poured into students who will demonstrate that they "have" them. The six Mindset Standards are well-intentioned:

> 1) Belief in development of whole self, including healthy balance of mental, social/emotional and physical well-being, 2) Self-confidence in ability to succeed, 3) Sense of belonging in the school environment, 4) Understanding postsecondary education and life-long learning are necessary for long-term career success, 5) Belief in using abilities to their fullest to achieve high-quality results and outcomes, 6) Positive attitude toward work and learning.
>
> (American School Counselor Association, 2014)

The ASCA Mindset notions have utility and could be reinterpreted in new ways. Each of these ASCA Mindset Standards could be shifted into a school community conversation that asks students, parents, and faculty specific questions. For instance, as part of a youth focus group or a Youth Participatory Action Research (YPAR) project, the Mindset Standards could be investigated and interrogated in terms of how they exist in the school community discourse and enactments:

1. How well do your teachers, administrators, and counselors foster the development of your whole self, including a healthy balance of mental, social/emotional, and physical well-being? Obviously, constructs such as "whole self" and "healthy balance" would have to be defined and interrogated by or with the students as part of a dialogical process.
2. How well do your teachers, administrators, and counselors foster your self-confidence and ability to succeed? What could they do

differently to help boost your self-confidence and ability to succeed? Is there an adult on campus you see as a self-confidence and ability booster for you?

3. How well do your teachers, administrators, and counselors foster your sense of belonging at our school? Are you part of a club or activity that makes you feel more connected to others at our school? Do you have suggestions for helping all students have a sense of belonging?

4. How well do your teachers, administrators, and counselors foster your understanding of postsecondary education and life-long learning as necessary for long-term career success? Do you know what you want to do after high school? Do you think you have enough information to get there? If not, do you know who to ask or where to get information that will help you meet your long-term goals?

5. How well do your teachers, administrators, and counselors believe you have the understanding and abilities to achieve your dreams?

6. How well are your teachers, administrators, and counselors fostering a positive attitude toward work and learning? Who does the best job of promoting students' positive attitudes toward work and learning?

As framed here, lifescaping mindsets are fostered in discourse. Discourses take place in relationships within the family, classroom, school, community, etc. The hope in schools is that individuals are invited to become active and engaged participants in discourses that foster growth and life-enhancing mindsets. In lifescaping, the hope is that we engage in dialogues that promote growth mindset discourses in our departments, schools, and communities.

In the eco-relational perspective undergirding lifescaping, individuals are understood as existing as members of family, classroom, school, and community ecologies. Let us briefly consider the individual constructs of both "mind" and "self" in connection to relationship. Siegel (2010) defines mind this way: "The human mind is a relational and embodied process that regulates the flow of energy and information" (p. 52). The point here is that mind is a relational process, and not isolated. In terms of self, Siegel (2012) states, "the idea of a unitary, continuous 'self' is actually an illusion our minds attempt to create . . . We have multiple and varied 'selves,' which are needed to carry out the many and diverse activities of our lives" (p. 229). The eco-relational perspective embraces the notion that our minds are a "relational and embodied process" and our "selves" are dependent upon the relationship contexts where we find ourselves. Thus, our relational history and current relational context influence how our current "self" is organized in the moment. The discourses we are engaged in shape who we are in the moment and the relational lifescapes we envision and make an effort to create. Relational understanding of "self" can encompass Naess' (1988) assertion regarding the need to cultivate an "ecological self" that encompasses the ecosystems and environment where we dwell as part of our "self-realization." Given the scale of the crisis of global warming, cultivating an eco-relational or ecological self may be necessary for human survival. In lifescaping, eco-relational understanding opens new possibilities for relationships with other people and the world where we dwell.

In lifescaping we accept responsibility for creating the life we live in relationship to everything around us; for those reading this book, we become teachers, counselors, psychologists, social workers, and administrators—educators all—in the hope we can create school communities where lifescaping is concerned with enhancing learning, well-being, and capacity to play for all students. Lifescaping becomes a form of learning that enriches our communities where we practice our professional craft and advocate for developing vibrant learning communities. We are driven by a desire to integrate lifescaping, well-being, and learning in schools in order to create just and compassionate communities of practice where human development flourishes.

Lifescaping Hope

Hope shapes and defines what we do with our careers and drives what we do to help others (Lewis, 2000). Even if the situation is logically hopeless, it is important to recognize that is when novelty and creativity come into play (Morin & Kern, 1999). Hope is not quiet and passive, or reserved for the comfortable middle-class or privileged elite, living alone in the forest. Hope is grounded in resilience and the recognition that suffering and struggle for survival do not diminish the capacity for human creativity and the desire to live a vibrant life with others. Paulo Freire (1997) asserts that hope is the ground that helps us to struggle for social justice; he stresses that we must have an education in hope. The activist writer Solnit says "hope is an ax you break down doors with in an emergency . . . Hope calls for action; action is impossible without hope" (2006, p. 5). Joanna Macy and Chris Johnstone (2012) offer tools for cultivating active hope as a practice that is exercised by bringing about what is hoped for. In this book we take the position that we live at a time when collective hope is required in our culture, and it is important to trust sources that foster and nurture our hope in lifescaping action taken in the struggle to create just and compassionate schools for all. Hope is tied to future forming and lifescaping; actions that are tied to the optimism that efforts will bear fruit. The ecology of action is a wager growing from hope; a bet where there is an awareness of the risks, the need to have a strategy that allows for modification, and even stopping the action if there are unforeseen consequences (Morin & Kern, 1999). Braidotti (2013) asserts, "Hope is a way of dreaming up possible futures: an anticipatory virtue that permeates our lives and activates them. It is a powerful motivating force grounded . . . in projects that aim at reconstructing the social imaginary" (p. 192). Hope connected to lifescaping can be directed toward creating a just and compassionate learning community where we find ourselves. Hope that informs and guides our lifescaping implies taking risks beyond what is given and what is comfortable for us individually; the struggles in the past fifty years by African-Americans, Native-Americans, Latino-Americans, LGBQT, and numerous other marginalized groups grew from the lifescaping hope of people determined to be heard and determined to have their voices listened to, needs addressed, and lives respected. The Norwegian philosopher Arne Naess (2002) points out, "One should not wander about and merely hope that things will turn out well; one ought to do something about it . . . Either we do something to realize our hopes, or we do what is useful *today*" (p. 167, italics in original).

Lifescaping hope directed at creating just and compassionate learning communities means having the courage to act by taking risks beyond what is given and what is comfortable, as well as beyond any notion of pre-conceived and packaged interventions. Lifescaping hope is having the courage to continue the struggle. Kenneth Gergen (2015) wonders, "Metaphorically speaking, what if we closed our eyes and began to imagine the worlds of our hopes? . . . what kind of world would we build?" (p. 6). The hope driving this text is that what is offered to you provides understandings to develop the know-how in lifescaping a more vibrant future for schools that is to become. Our hope is that "seeing with new eyes" will incite resistance to the status quo, press researchers to attempt to build or create new "forms of life" in their local schools and to create communities of practice concerned with the enhancement of the well-being of all (Gergen, 2015). The future forming and lifescaping practices described in this text offer maps, but readers should always bear in mind that any map is not the territory.

This book is meant to serve as a guide to using an engaged strengths-based eco-relational process in creative inquiry directed toward promoting relational wellness, learning power, and reflective action on behalf of and with students in schools understood as learning communities. The text orients readers to a strengths-based, eco-relational and participatory framework (e.g., Galassi & Akos, 2007; Lewis & Borunda, 2006; Naess, 2002; Skolimowski, 1994). The book is designed to guide student advocates (school helping professionals and community members) inter-ested in successful "actionability" and in creating the "relational moment" where they know they are in it together (Gergen, 2006). That is to say, this is a book for those who are interested in lifescaping in their unique school community; it offers pathways for asserting agency in the unfolding relational moment, your home life, and in the here-and-now—or living moment. Like artistic attempts to bring awe and appreciation to landscapes, lifescaping attempts to evoke hope, curiosity, illumination, connection, compassion, play, and a burning desire to take action to bring the moment into full light and expression, etc. When considering lifescaping, personal agency, dramatic engagement, successful action, and enhancing the relational moment are crucial; as is living with a "solar ethic" where, like the sun, one burns brightly with energy and expressive life (Cupitt, 1995). Think about your hopes, actions, and desire to make a positive connection on a first date with someone you are excited to be going out with, or with someone you really value and want to create a growing relationship with; agency is required to ask, the story in your head moves dramatically toward your desired goal, and your actions are focused on creating the relational moment where you both feel connected to each other in new and life-affirming ways.

Success and the relational moment are achieved by enacting excellence in practice; which means the necessity to reflect upon and adjust practice in light of achieved results occurring in lived contexts beyond the dialogue in your head, consulting room, classroom or college lecture hall. Excellence is aspirational and tapped into when individuals are in *flow*, a conscious state experienced when fully engaged in an activity that demands skill and know-how that emerge as self-confidence, competence, and total focus on what is being done in the moment (Csikszentmihalyi, 1990). Flow can happen (but not always) when individuals engage in activities that evoke love and passion, such as playing music, rock climbing, doing tai chi, counseling, teaching, leading a community meeting, etc. Experiencing flow in any of these activities is not a given and not a guaranteed experience. Yet, flow is always possible when individuals and groups focus themselves in a manner that opens them up to playfully utilizing skilled know-how and energy engaged in the task at hand; flow can also be related to "vital engagement" or loving what one is doing (Haidt, 2006, p. 224). Flow can be connected to Goleman's "focus" construct (2013). We assert that flow is fostered by cultivating performative focus discourses linked to Vygotsky's (1986) "zone of proximal development," the gap between our current level and potential level of development via play. Play flows, especially for children, where they learn to perform being who they are not (a make believe Mommy, Daddy, doctor or pirate). In play, we learn to create new forms of life for ourselves and our friends in ways that flow. Play that flows liberates us from ways of being that oppress or hold us back to "the way things are." Play activity that flows has value because we free ourselves to become the producers, builders, and creators of our lives in the moment. We learn to become producers, builders, and creators by playfully engaging in lifescaping and future forming actions. Coupled with the flow that comes from free play, we also learn from more knowledgeable others and the scaffolding they offer helps us as learners navigate between the boredom of routine tasks and the anxiety of not having a clue. Having mentors, coaches, and allies who connect learning with play fosters our ability to engage in activities linked to flow.

Flow is not something that emerges merely from the environment or the person; in this text flow is framed as relational—emerging in the interaction between the person and task; flow emerges as a result of the relationships and actions taking place, not from the lecture, text, armchair, or plan. Joy, identity, and connectedness emerge from focused engagement in doing the task at hand in the moment; time and action become fused in concentrated activity directed toward specific goals. Flow is not the text, but the composing moment where the action is in the world, engaged with others, or even in becoming totally engaged in doing something alone.

We teach and counsel others. Sometimes there is flow. Other times the lessons taught are not the lessons learned. Teaching is relational and is best when the process is concentrated on doing/reflection, which can exist in reading, math, science, art, counseling, or car repair. Counseling is relational and best when concerned with doing/reflection, such as focusing the therapeutic conversation on helping clients achieve personally meaningful goals, which can be doing/reflection decision making, taking steps toward goals, listening, and, rather recursively, improving relationships and thinking about thinking. Doing/reflection is taking action and assessing results. Doing/reflection can concentrate on course content or perceptions of competence and specialness; doing/reflection is best if it is tied to engaging in something that is meaningful to individuals, where they can experience vital engagement, love for what they are engaged in, and flow. Sometimes an important lesson focuses on teaching students with little faith in their abilities the steps necessary to recognize and tap their competence and power. It is vital to cultivate compassion for learners and for oneself as a helper in this life flow (Gilbert, 2009).

As an advocate, it is important to remain humble and listen deeply to students, parents, colleagues, and others to enter their world to understand and empathize with their experience, values, desires, and goals. If our goal is to support all students to develop "twenty-first century" skills and capacities, then deep and active engagement of helping professionals and other school community members is critical. We want to create strengths-based school ecologies where the community discourse cultivates "co-vitality," the co-occurrence of multiple positive psychological traits (Furlong, You, Renshaw, Smith, & O'Malley, 2013; Renshaw et al., 2014).

The strengths-based eco-relational approach described in this book integrates relational, developmental, dialogical, interactional, meaning making, narrative, and strengths-based practices concentrated on doing/reflection, which are actions (e.g., Bronfenbrenner, 1979; Bruner, 1986, 1990, 1996, 2002; Buber, 1970; Capra, 2002; Claxton, 1999, 2002; Conyne & Cook, 2004; Cooperrider & Whitney, 2005; Furlong et al., 2013; Galassi & Akos, 2007; Gergen, 2009; Goleman et al., 2012; Lewis, 2011; Lewis & Hatch, 2008; Linell, 2009; Mehl-Madrona, 2010; Monk, Winslade, Crocket, & Epston, 1997; Myers & Sweeney, 2005; Paisley & Hubbard, 1994; Peavy, 2004; Prilleltensky & Prilleltensky, 2005, 2006; Reason & Bradbury, 2008; Reese & Myers, 2012; Renshaw et al., 2014; Skolimowski, 1994; Smith, 1975, 1982, 1986, 2006; Smith & Williams, 1999; Sterling, 2001).

Humans are citizens of the web of life, and participants in a beautiful and sometimes terrifying world and universe. As participants and members in a living planetary existence, humans have a responsibility to each other and the life systems they belong to. A strengths-based eco-relational approach draws upon our collective sense of responsibility to and for one another as we are called upon to better serve our youth, our students. The desire to better serve students fuels participatory inquiry within schools.

Leading Participatory Inquiry

Pedro Noguera's notion of "critical supporters" guides Peg's work with leaders of participatory inquiry. Noguera (2003) describes critical supporters as those who recognize the education rights of children and their parents and thus demonstrate active support for change and improvement. Peg extends this definition as she guides leaders not to speak for others, but rather to engage marginalized families (and community members) in the discourse so they become the critical supporters. Advocates must nurture an environment and a process open to considering a variety of strategies for innovation. In keeping with Noguera's work, inquiry must move beyond a blind embrace of the latest educational reform bandwagon, as participants must honestly identify what is not working for students and pursue actions to address failings at a school. Critical supporters assess reforms based not only on students' academic outcomes, but also on the learning community experience described by students and their families. This is an inherently collaborative, not "top down" approach to school improvement.

Lewis and Borunda (2006) define participatory leadership as leadership that emerges from engagement and participation in collaborative efforts to bring about systemic change in specific schools by advocating for all students, especially those who have been traditionally marginalized. Participatory leadership does not require a big hat or a big title because it emerges from one's ethical and moral positioning. Participatory leadership requires the skills necessary to advocate that nurturing relationships with individuals, groups, other stakeholders, and most of all, students should engage school communities in constructing democratic institutions where the challenges facing communities can be addressed directly by those involved. Students, parents, staff, teachers, counselors, school psychologists, administrators—all school community members—are capable of exploring the positive core of the school community and building on it. Participatory leadership is a form of leadership that is shared among helping professionals in schools, districts, and organizations in promoting a more just and democratic society. This requires that professionals give up the idea that there is an elite group of highly trained philosopher-kings, similar to those in Plato's *Republic*, who are the interpreters and custodians of some hidden truth or a singular answer. Participatory leadership requires that professionals move beyond talk of being saved by motivational speakers or other fashionable messianic leaders and toward becoming empowered participatory and local leaders who bring diverse voices that focus on how and what works to help all students in local communities and contexts thrive, and draw upon deep democratic traditions that emerge from a simple principle: *e pluribus unum*. School administrators must have the skill and the will to embrace participatory leadership and include diverse voices in decisions at their sites. Often community members, other than the site administrator, have the skills and relationships to facilitate participatory inquiry. Thus site administrators must serve—and encourage others to serve—as participatory leaders within the school and district community. As advocates, we are mindful of how and why we engage in participatory inquiry regardless of who is leading a particular focus group, planning meeting, event or action.

Advocacy, Action and Reflection: We See, We Hear, We Are Not Quiet about What We See and Hear

A long time ago, someone shared a quote with Rolla but he forgets who that someone was, and now the quote floats around his mind like so many other important sources of wisdom that emerge in conversation with the company he keeps. He shares this not to confess about his fading memory, but to speak about how much of what we carry, especially the wisdom, comes from conversations and contact with the people we talk to, hang around with at work, home, and in transit. Although a digression, this is shared in order to point out that schools are communities where kids are compelled to hang around with people who might teach them to love learning or teach them to run away from the lesson at hand (Smith, 1998). Still, to be human is to be learning. Humans learn regardless of the lesson taught. Ultimately, we learn on our own or with others, and hopefully, we learn how to live in the fullest sense of our greater humanity, however that is defined. To be human is to be using language and telling stories to others in our family, group, club, or gang that help us make sense of being in this world at certain moments in time (Boyd, 2009; Britton, 1970; Claxton, 1999, 2002; Mehl-Madrona, 2010; Smith, 1975, 2006). That is why certain things seem to linger with us.

Back to the quote: although the reference is lost to Rolla, the quote is attributed to Jose Saramargo, who was awarded the 1998 Nobel Prize for literature. Rolla was told (notice the linguistic gambit toward telling a story rather than offering a reference; such is everyday memory and story), Saramargo said that three things define our humanity: one, we can see; two, we can hear; and three, we do not have to be quiet or complacent about what we see and hear. Rolla likes that quote and has used it to inform his work as a counselor educator, professor, and teacher because it is about advocacy in education. The quote offers a seed idea that is connected to democracy, narrative, action, the participatory inquiry process, and the appreciative inquiry process that are expanded on later in this text. This work draws upon the wisdom inherent in the following points:

1. *We can see.* In this book you will be given some tools for looking at your school. You will look at the physical environment, the building, the classrooms, hallways, and bathrooms. You will look at how people treat and relate to and play with each other. You will look at the data regarding test scores, absences, tardiness, fights, violence, bullying, and any other data that will enable you to see how the school is currently operating in order to improve capacity as a learning community. You will look at your community, school (students, faculty, staff, and administration), and group demographics.

2. *We can hear.* You will listen to teachers, counselors, administrators, parents, students, and other community members about their experience in the school. The important point here is not to jump to conclusions but to listen, to understand that schools are filled with multiple stories where some stories will dominate and even silence other valid and alternative stories. Listen to every person's story, as a certain point of view rather than some unquestionable Truth that can rule out other people's stories. Like all communities and organizations, schools have many voices and stories. It will be particularly important for you to seek the stories of school community members from historically marginalized populations. Systems reproduce themselves and those who have power will continue to have power and those who struggle will continue to struggle unless we intentionally disrupt the stories being cycled through the engagement and inclusion of under-represented perspectives. Your job is to explore how to give the diverse voices opportunity to be heard in a community of multiple voices. Listen intently to the relational flow between and among individuals and groups in your school community. You will hear how many different individuals' stories are told to make sense and meaning from their experience being in the same school community.

3. *We are not quiet about what we see and hear.* Knowing how not to be quiet is an art. There are times to shout and there are times to calmly press for change. Shouting at the right time may save an individual or change a community. Shouting at the wrong time may result in trauma to the community or marginalize and even hurt individuals. Calmly and courageously pressing for change may result in swift change or may result in years of effort to move an organization and community (Hatch & Lewis, 2011). We need to speak, but we also need to listen deeply. We best serve our communities when we create a space for those who have not been heard, to be heard and engaged in the process of change. We aspire to speak with, not for, those who are under-served.

4. *We take action as advocates.* Advocacy is not easy. Advocacy calls for mindfulness and even *mindful wonder*—which is a curiosity, wonder, and awe about what is being said by students, colleagues, and others working within the organization (Lewis, Lenski, Mukhopadhyay, & Cartwright, 2010). Advocacy calls for exceptional relational skills that invite all parties to engage in respectful dialogue (Bemak & Chung, 2005; Lee, 2007; Ratts, DeKruyf, & Chen-Hayes, 2007). Advocacy calls for compassion and empathy for difference (Gilbert, 2009). The counseling profession has defined advocacy competencies that can help guide practice. Counselors are encouraged to review and become familiar with the advocacy competencies (see Lewis, Arnold, House, & Toporek, 2002; also, http://counseling.org/resources/). The expectations for advocacy are embedded in the California Professional Standards for Educational Leadership, CPSELs. School leaders must navigate and advocate even as they name and frame their work. For instance, while school leaders are consistently challenged to close the "achievement gap," the term opportunity gap more accurately describes current schooling practices. We view social justice as an essential advocacy principle. In the words of Lindsey, Lindsey, & Terrell (2011), "Social justice moves leaders from awareness to *action*, from skill to *will*, from them to *us*, and from then to *now!*" (p. 42).

   Life is a stage, and schools are local theaters where advocates engage in ethical enactments that are geared toward helping all students tap their relational wellness and learning power. In this book, work to understand and appreciate your relationships with others in your school setting, and make use of what is going to help you take action to improve your school or enhance your professional skills. Advocacy is part of this.

5. *We reflect deeply upon the impact of our actions.* In reflecting, we recognize that some actions have unintended consequences that we cannot foresee. We respond to those and continue to collaboratively construct the future we want to build in the schools where we are. Set aside what is not working and come back later when you are ready to make alternative decisions about what does not vitally engage you. If possible, let go of those things that have no meaning to you as you move forward into your life and career; this work is driven by vital engagement and a growth mindset.

As an advocate you may serve—or encourage others to serve—as leaders of inquiry. As you move through a participatory inquiry process at your site you will want to notice and reflect upon your own responses before posing questions to other community members. We want to take reflective moments.

Reflective Moment 1.1

Please take the time to write a response to the following questions in order to clarify, shape, and define your own thinking about the questions and perspective being raised and forwarded in this text around what you see and hear.

- In your current school or professional setting, how are you (as an individual and a professional) acting toward other members of your community in this moment?
- Are you listening to what is being said (by students, clients, colleagues, parents, and others) or focused on making some point of your own?
- In this present moment, are there possibilities for dialogue, where you can listen to and respond to individuals and members of a group? How well are you listening? Do you really understand the other person's story from their perspective? How well can you summarize what they have shared?
- What ecological elements are contributing to your own responses or actions?

Reflective Moment 1.2

Please take the time to write your responses to the following questions in order to define your own thinking about the questions and the perspective being raised in this text. Consider the implications of your responses for the students you serve as a professional and how you might use some of these questions and responses in facilitating the participatory inquiry process.

Here are some questions advocates should ask themselves if they are not going to be quiet about what they see and hear:

- What are one or two things you/we are doing to foster positive and supportive relationships with colleagues, among students, parents, and community members?
- What are one or two things you/we are doing to foster student or collegial wellness?
- How do you/we take part in socializing yourself/ourselves into not seeing issues of inequity in your/our community?
- Do you/we feel helping professionals (school counselors, school psychologists, school administrators, and other educators) are functionaries of the existing educational structures? If so, how so?

- How can you/we as student advocates (school counselors, school psychologists, school administrators, and other educators) act to support all students to find their own sense of competence where their potential and talents will be fostered by adults who provide care and support, define high expectations, and create opportunities for kids to participate in activities they find meaningful (Benard, 2004; Brooks & Goldstein, 2001; Hatch & Lewis, 2011)?

Chapter Summary

This chapter provides a philosophical and conceptual foundation for the rest of the book. It offers a strengths-based ecological perspective that is directed toward making schools vibrant learning communities. The chapter introduces the notions of both future forming and lifescaping as actions moving and shaping the discourse and learning environment by people living and working in those schools. The act of lifescaping requires engagement in enacting social justice as a form of education in hope. Lifescaping requires courage, the recognition that practitioners must endeavor to find flow by navigating between the boredom of the given and the anxiety of the unknown. Such courage requires new forms of leadership. The chapter offers participatory leadership, leaders who do not wear the big hat, but leaders who invite collaboration and inclusion as ways of leading participatory inquiry directed toward lifescaping practices in their schools. Leaders are school administrators, counselors, psychologists, social workers, teachers, and other community members who advocate for youth. These advocates see, hear, and speak out about what they see and hear; they also take action and reflect upon the impact of those actions. They continually engage in lifescaping in their learning communities.

2 Relational Ecosystems and Learning Power in Schools

We come to conceive of a "real world" in a manner that fits the stories we tell about it, but it is our good philosophical fortune that we are forever tempted to tell different stories about the presumably same events in the presumably real world. The tyranny of the single story surely led our forebears to guarantee freedom of expression, as in the First Amendment to the United States Constitution. Let many stories bloom.

(Jerome Bruner, 2002, p. 103)

A human being is part of a whole, called by us "Universe," a part limited in time and space. He [sic] experiences himself, his thoughts and feelings, as something separated from the rest—a kind of optical delusion of his consciousness . . .

(Albert Einstein, 1950)

Relational Ecosystems

From Bronfenbrenner's (1979) ecological perspective, individuals and groups are always viewed as existing within ecosystemic contexts. We exist in biological ecologies and social ecologies immersed in eco-relationships. We find ourselves in human and biological ecological niches, life patterns, life spaces, and eco-relationships where life narratives are told. People exist in ecosystems, which are the interlocking influences operating at all levels of human life, from the individual, family, community, state, nation, world in terms of human ecosystems, and from the soil, plants, air, and entire life system in terms of the ecosystems where all life exits. Humans are not separate; human ecosystems are nested within life ecosystems that constitute a living ecosphere teeming with eco-relationships (see Appendix B).

People have their own chronological lived moment set in a particular time, social, and ecological context. Individuals exist in ecological niches where the various aspects of the ecosystem regularly influence their eco-relational life pattern and life space (Conyne & Cook, 2004). The *ecological niche* is where the person lives, the place, such as urban, rural, United States, Mexico, etc. The person's *life pattern* describes the why of their life. Such as, why does this person live in a rural area? Why does this person shop at the farmer's market or Wal-Mart? Thus, life pattern is made up of internal and external elements. Whereas, *life space* is defined by the combination of ecological niche and life pattern (Conyne & Cook, 2004). Life space gets at the internal and external elements that make up a person's life, and may be mapped eco-relationally with individuals (Peavy, 2004). For instance, a new third-grade student moves into a rural school district (niche) because his parents are migrant farmworkers who have fled Mexico to escape the violence induced by cartels fighting over turf in their village (life pattern). In working with the child a counselor explores the child's life space by creating a life map. The life map might reveal a complicated *life narrative* and eco-relational connections related to the family's flight from the community violence prompted unintentionally by the U.S. war on drugs and by the regional Mexican cartel trying to get their products to a high-demand U.S. black-market. The example is meant to show that individuals are always nested eco-relationally in multiple systems. In working with such a student, it would be helpful to understand their ecological niche, life pattern, life space, life narrative, and eco-relationships as much as possible. If there is more than one individual and even a group of students with similar life space stories, advocates should consider developing specific strategies and support systems to create a life space in the school community that enhances and promotes the eco-relationships and learning for those students.

We are all in a certain *flow of life* where we must become aware of ourselves as actors in a drama involving all living beings who seek to reduce their own suffering, maximize their happiness, maintain their health, and learn to live with ease, elegance, and grace (Gilbert, 2009). The flow of life defines our eco-relational lifescapes and lifescaping efforts.

Embedded Self and Relational Responsibilities

Eco-relational counseling in schools views people as participating agents embedded within interlocking social systems, or social ecologies (Bronfenbrenner, 1979; Conyne & Cook, 2004; Goleman et al., 2012; Lewis, 2011; Prilleltensky & Prilleltensky, 2006; Skolimowski, 1994; Sterling, 2001). Additionally, humans are also part of interlocking life systems that include air, water, earth, and animals; our common ecosystems are our life-community to which we all belong (Bowers, 1997, 2003; Capra, 2002; Goleman et al., 2012; Leopold, 1949; Spretnak, 2011; Williams & Brown, 2012). Understanding social and bio-ecological connectedness is crucial; people are part of, not separate from, the life systems they are embedded in and surrounded by. Humans participate as members of a living planet and as agents in human life-communities (Bowers, 1997, 2000; Capra, 1996, 2002; Goleman et al., 2012; Leopold, 1949; Skolimowski, 1994; Spretnak, 2011; Sterling, 2001; Williams & Brown, 2012). Although much of the work in schools concentrates on the interactions between people and human systems, ecological counseling in the schools is a heuristic grounded in and taking an active role in linking personal, social, academic, and career education to promoting sustainable ecological health and wellness.

Merely talking about and taking action in the human and social ecology is not enough. People breathe the air and exist as part of the land and biological systems that surround them. The notion seems obvious, but individualism in the United States seems to foster the belief that a lone cowboy or cowgirl can make his or her way as separate and above the hostile world where they travel outside of any authentic relationship with other people or the landscape. The point here is not to imply any criticism of personal initiative, but to recognize that humans are not separate isolated entities that can be set apart from social and biological systems. Humans are part of and citizens of social and biological systems and ecologies; individual selves are not separated, regardless of any myths or personal existential fears. In fact, Naess (1988, 2002) asserts that self-realization is tied to seeing oneself as part of the larger social and biological ecology where people exist as living beings.

People live out a sense of self intimately connected to the kinds of social conditions in which they are embedded and in the dialogues they engage in (Linell, 2009). Linell argues the self is dialogical and embedded in social and biological contexts, connections, and interconnections. In fact, the dialogical view sees the self as constantly in flux, constantly changing depending upon the dialogues and relationships the person is engaged in throughout their life. In other words, individual meaning moves; meaning is never fixed; it is relational, evolving, and subject to critical reflection. As such, meaning is always contestable, and different, alternative meanings are possible (Dragonas, Gergen, McNamee, & Tselious, 2015; Gergen, 2009; Linell, 2009; Peavy, 2004). This points to how our lifescapes are fluid and our lifescaping efforts and actions have the possibility of shifting in new directions.

Human identity becomes thoroughly relational; dialogue and agency become pathways for taking truth out from inside the heads of individuals and into the negotiated space between persons in communities (Isaacs, 1999; Linell, 2009; Peavy, 2004). The words we use do not spring from our heads, we are born into evolving languages that we learn in families, communities, and cultures; the languages we speak existed here long before we did, as did the biological and ecological communities where we were raised. As advocates, action becomes less bound in individual heroics and more concerned with fostering the potential for relationships, dialogue, and coordinated actions that can build, sustain, and evolve with learning communities and lifescapes over time.

As student advocates, it is important to recognize that *relationships* (social and biological) are everything in life; *participation* is the glue that connects individuals to each other, their families, schools, communities, and ecosystems; *action* informs and transforms relationships and participation throughout the social and biological living systems where people exist. Each individual and group can foster positive relationships, participate more fully, and take action to inform and transform or support the systems where they exist. How we frame and story ourselves in those multiple roles impacts what we do. Hence, it is important for each of us as individuals to patch together knowledge and skills into heuristics that can help guide our actions and provide us with a sense of agency that we can teach and share within our community. Strengths-based ecological counseling in the schools is united with efforts to promote ecological well-being in communities and engage in participative lifescaping actions (Conyne & Cook, 2004; Galassi & Akos, 2007; Goleman et al., 2012; Kelly, 2000; Peavy, 2004; Prilleltensky & Prilleltensky, 2006; Reese & Myers, 2012; Skolimowski, 1994; Sterling, 2001).

The key characteristic in the approach taken in this text is that meaning-making in the human social web of life is linked to connectedness with the physical environment and the social environment; individuals, families, communities, nations, and the web of human life are viewed and understood within their earthen landscapes and the web of biological life. Action involves contextualized dialogues that are dependent on the meaning participants derive from their environmental interactions, both social and biological. The helping dialogue aims to assist and empower participants (as individuals, groups, and systems) to tap their wellness by increasing their agency and capacity to learn and enact life-enhancing and life-sustaining choices. Individuals are viewed as learning beings existing as part of and within families and communities set in local biological communities. Families, groups, and human communities are also viewed as being nested in biological ecosystems. Connectedness matters. Every word uttered and action taken involves the potential to learn about or enter more deeply into *relationships* (social and biological) that might enhance the lifespace. Gergen (2009) points to embracing *"relational responsibility"* as a way of replacing individual responsibility and blame (p. 364). Every word and action invites *participation* that significantly connects people to each other, their families, schools, communities, and life ecosystems. Every *action* teaches, informs, and has the power to transform relationships, one's sense of agency, and how individuals participate in the social and biological living systems where they exist. People exist in and take action in social, biological, and learning webs that define their lifescapes.

The Learning Power Construct

Schools are learning communities, for better or worse. Better for kids who flourish, and worse for kids who learn that school sucks. All advocates working in schools are essentially educators who focus on fostering the learning power of students. Advocates in the schools have an obligation to help all students live into their greatest potential academically, personally, socially, occupationally, and as contributing citizens in their school and community. Learning power is a term coined by Claxton (1999). Learning power is an active process that invites students to become engaged learners and agents by doing and learning about things that are meaningful to them, and by encouraging students to persist in learning things that are difficult (Claxton, 2002; Claxton et al., 2011). Encouragement, invitation, agency, and tenacity are part of learning power; it is about cultivating a growth mindset to overcome learning obstacles (Dweck, 2006). Mentoring, being an ally or coach, and creating opportunities for students to learn how to relate to each other as humans living life, as students, and as teachers fosters learning power. Learning power development emerges from how we relate to each other in exploring our possibilities and hopes, as well as our performative efforts to bring about the world we want to live in.

Tragically, talented teens are documented to become alienated from school when they fail to see connection and meaning in the lessons presented in classrooms (Csikszentmihalyi, Rathunde, Whalen, & Wong, 1993). According to results from the 2006–2008 California Healthy Kids Survey, in 472 districts and 1380 schools where 561,317 ninth and eleventh grade students were surveyed, fewer than 20 percent of all students indicated that they had high levels of meaningful participation at school. This is not the students' fault; this is a systemic failure. Since the 1980s fear has dominated the educational discourse, and public education and educators have become scapegoats for the problems plaguing society. *A nation at risk* (National Commission on Excellence in Education, 1983) reported test scores of U.S. students on national and international scales and raised public concern about the perceived decline of academic achievement in the United States. Response to the report did not take into account the large percentage of American youth engaged in public education and the inclusion of children who might not receive a public education in other countries (or in earlier decades in the U.S.). Politicians addressed public anxiety about the educational system by legislating No Child Left Behind (NCLB) in 2001 (U.S. Department of Education, 2002). NCLB focused on the so-called achievement gap, revealing race and class achievement differences in standardized test scores. The response was to test, re-test, and to punish schools that did not improve test scores, rather than figuring out how to engage and invite students into developing their learning power. The NCLB led to Race to the Top in 2009 (U.S. Department of Education, 2009) and policies that had different states and districts competing for limited educational funds. Teachers were evaluated based on students' test scores, schools that did not improve could have their principals fired, and other drastic measures were instituted.

Both NCLB and Race to the Top were driven by fear that U.S. students cannot compete in a global market. Race to the Top pitted states against each other in competition over funds to improve test scores and educational outcomes along the lines mandated by the federal government. The NCLB and Race to the Top school reforms are based on politics, not pedagogy. Both NCLB and Race to the Top were disasters that imposed oppressive demands on students, teachers, parents, and administrators (Ravitch, 2016). Both degraded public education, and led some critics to assert that educational policy in the United States is guided by "lifeless mechanistic metaphors" and market-driven practices (Williams & Brown, 2012, p. 5). Sadly, this notion of U.S. policy regarding education in the United States is consistent with Paul Goodman's (1960) criticism over fifty years ago where he asserted that in the United States students are growing up absurd. This sense of educational absurdity comes into focus with the student responses in the WestEd study. According to results from the 2006–2008 California Healthy Kids Survey reported by WestEd (2010), in 472 districts and 1380 schools where 561,317 ninth and eleventh grade students were surveyed, fewer than 20 percent of all students indicated that they had high levels of meaningful participation at school. The results reveal many kids learn that there is little meaningful participation in schools where poor and disenfranchised youth move along what is referred to as a school-to-prison pipeline. It is crucial to question the efficacy of school systems where over 30 percent of students do not succeed. The point is not to despair, but to recognize the need to advocate for schools to promote protective factors that enhance learning, where wisdom and sound educational practices invite students and educators to engage in meaningful activities that enhance the learning power of all (e.g., Adelman & Taylor, 2006a, 2006b; Chappuis, 2009; Chappuis, Stiggins, Arter, & Chappuis, 2005; Claxton, 1997, 1999, 2002, 2008; Comstock, 2005; Dewey, 1929/1960; Dragonas et al., 2015; Dweck, 2006; Finser, 2007; Goleman et al., 2012; Keltner, 2009; Paisley & Hubbard, 1994; Squier et al., 2014; Sterling, 2001; Stone, 2009; Williams & Brown, 2012).

As of 2015, the Every Student Succeeds Act (ESSA) replaced NCLB. Some critics refer to ESSA as the Everything Stays the Same Act because those who benefit most from such efforts are the educational reform industry, which makes billions from consulting and delivering services related to meeting ESSA mandates, and super-rich philanthropists who are both colonizing public schools with initiatives such as Bill Gates' Common Core agenda and dismantling public education by promoting school "choice" like the Walton family efforts (Au & Hollar, 2016). Some advocates are encouraging parents of color to revolt against standardized testing because of the reductionist way assessments are used to define the teaching curriculum by marginalizing the arts and other creative possibilities for students; thus, the obsession with standardized testing limits both the content being taught and the learning number of options for the children and youth to cultivate their potential and talents (Hagopian, 2016).

Time will tell how ESSA works or does not work, who profits from ESSA and who does not, but there may emerge opportunities for educators and parents who want to work at a local level to advocate for alternative measures of learning and development, such as electronic learning logs or portfolios. E-portfolios and learning logs enable students to save and keep their own exemplars of school work and projects over time, to document how their skills and knowledge have developed, to reflect on what they have learned, and to be able to share their learning and challenges with supportive educators who focus on building student learning power. Opting out of standardized testing and having students develop their own learning logs or portfolios is a real option in this internet age. Wakimoto and Lewis (2014) share how such electronic professional practice portfolios (ePPP) are used with graduate students on a free and accessible platform; the same tools could be used to create inexpensive electronic platforms for students to develop learning portfolios they could access and take with them regardless of the school they attended. What ESSA becomes will depend on how effectively professionals and communities advocate for genuine engagement in learning and control over local schools. The push in this text is to shout out that action research is a tool for documenting efforts in local schools to help every student succeed. The action research and participatory inquiry promoted in this text can be aligned with ESSA's mandate for documenting local efforts to help every student succeed.

Years ago, E. F. Schumacher (1973) asserted that education could become a destructive force if it does not clarify students' central convictions rather than merely trying to meet the instrumental needs of the market place. Indeed, there is a public purpose for education where students are invited to participate in civic engagement and shown how sustaining an energetic democracy depends upon citizens who live up to certain civic responsibilities (Goodlad & McMannon, 1997). Schools would be better served if there was more concentration on promoting learning power by assessing *for* learning in order to help students understand that to be human is to be learning (Chappuis, 2009; Chappuis et al., 2005). Helping students appreciate their agency and learning power is vital for maintaining any true democracy. Sadly, this text does not have space to explore and develop the criticism more deeply. This text offers the participatory inquiry process as a vehicle to enhance the lives of students, the vitality of professionals, and the community where they find themselves.

This book taps into the metaphors of fostering academic (head), personal/social (heart), and work/career (hands) development (Hatch & Lewis, 2011). It is important to integrate teaching head, heart, and hands (3-H) in schools without pitting abstract knowledge against practical knowledge (Bowers, 2000; Gandhi, 1953; Goleman et al., 2012; Hatch & Lewis, 2011; Williams & Brown, 2012). We have known for a very long time that students learn via experience (Archambault, 1964; Dewey, 1938); by being engaged in doing things that are meaningful to them, both in the abstract sense of sticking to math in order to become an engineer, and the practical sense of learning how automotive engines work in order to repair them. The important concern is making sure that students graduate from high school with a sense of competence in knowing what they know as learners and as citizens, as well as the resilience and resourcefulness to face the unknown and other challenges that are part of living in this world. Dewey (1929/1960) argued long ago that a culture that believes in freedom needs to believe in education. Further, education should help cultivate citizens who are growing, reflective, thoughtful, and inquiring agents in their lives and communities. The developmental perspective, reflective practice, mindfulness, and curiosity promoted throughout this book align with Dewey what was asserting early in the twentieth century. Education is a cornerstone for any functioning democracy.

The eco-relational view espoused in the text sees knowledge as cultivated and maintained socially. "Knowledge is seen not as something that a person *has* (or does not have), but as something that people *do* together" (Burr, 1995, p. 8). Behavior and learning are interactional and dynamic; people come into being interacting with their environment, which is a network or meshwork of each other and the world around them (Conyne & Cook, 2004). Interdependence and mutuality are "central to psychological growth and emotional and physical well-being" (Comstock, 2005, p. xiv).

Reflective Moment 2.1

Please take the time to write your responses to the following questions in order to define your own thinking about the questions and the perspective being raised in this text. Consider the implications of your responses for the students you serve as a professional and how you might use some of these questions and responses in facilitating the participatory inquiry process.

Here are some questions to consider in exploring your own ecological context and the ecological context of your students:

- Describe an *ecological niche* where you find yourself. What is your *life pattern* emerging from this niche? What is your *life space*? Briefly write a one paragraph life narrative that integrates your ecological niche, life pattern, and life space.
- Practice the above exercise with a student. You will have to orient them to the terms or change them to fit your relationship with the student.

Here are some questions advocates should ask themselves about learning power:

- Give your own definition of learning power. How has your own learning power impacted your life?
- How have you fostered the learning power of others?
- How has your learning and development been fostered by your relationship with others?
- How are relationships, participation, and action tied to learning power?
- How are learning and doing connected in your own life?
- How can you foster and promote the learning power and success of all students at our school?

Connecting Chapters 1 and 2:

- What are one or two things you/we are doing to encourage students or colleagues to develop their learning power, an active process focused on vital engagement and doing things that are meaningful to learners while fostering their academic (head), personal/social (heart), and work/career (hands) development?

Chapter Summary

This chapter expands on the relational nature of the strengths-based eco-relational perspective by exploring relational ecosystems. The chapter deepens our understanding of how we are all connected and related, and how our selves are formed in relationships, not in isolation. It then links relationships to Guy Claxton's learning power construct and the need to foster learning power in all students. The chapter asserts that the 2015 Every Student Succeeds Act (ESSA) could be used as an opportunity for school districts to use action research and appreciative inquiry to find out what works to help foster students' learning power in their local schools. As forms of future forming and lifescaping assessments, both action research and appreciative inquiry could be promoted in schools to demonstrate what they are doing to ensure that every student succeeds. Those efforts could also be used to define what students are going to succeed at doing, learning, and living in the school community.

3 Nurturing Growth Narratives in School Communities

Knowledge is not like a pile of bricks which, when it becomes large enough, magically turns into a house; it is like a tree that grows by daring to put out shoots into the unknown.

(Guy Claxton and Bill Lucas, 2015, p. 29)

Education becomes an open inquiry into what works when we engage in a continuing conversation and deep practice about how to work together in sustaining a learning community. An effective learning community invites educators and students to collaborate in ways that engage both in achieving some end, be it teaching–learning of Geometry or producing a school musical performance. Care and support, high expectations, and meaningful participation are balanced and guide practice (Benard, 2004). The meaning students derive emerges from the ongoing dialogue and conversations with those around them, both in school and out of school (Conyne & Cook, 2004; Linell, 2009). Community and student "truth" varies historically and cross-culturally according to the stories told and what works in a given context. Current accepted ways of under-standing the world are products of social processes, interactions, dialogues, and stories in which people are constantly engaged with each other. Truth becomes what works and hangs together in the best possible way in the community where you live (Boyd, 2009; Dewey, 1929/1960; Hayes, Hayes, Reese, & Sarbin, 1993). "What works" is storied, relational, and dialogi-cal; successful students figure out the many landmarks to follow while moving through the learning environment.

"What works" should always be interrogated. Otherwise a complicity about "what is" emerges, and the lifescape begins to look static and stuck rather than as a fluid human construct, like a garden. Sometimes it is necessary to replace a plant or redesign an area of the garden. In school communities, some members have louder voices than others, and it is important to listen and actively seek the stories of students and parents who are not being served or heard. Advocates engage in making what works inclusive of all voices and making sure there are active efforts to solicit the diverse voices in the community. Thus, open inquiry must interrogate preferred and privileged narratives that might silence others; this is especially important in schools where there are large numbers of dropouts (or push outs), low achievement, and other indicators of community withdrawal from school as an institution that cultivates student potential. Failing schools are framed as part of a school-to-prison pipeline, not as learning communities.

Recognizing and Interrogating Privileged Narratives in Schools

While education is frequently and inappropriately proposed as the "cure" or at least as a treatment to heal the gravest ills of society (i.e. poverty), schools operate as microsystems, mirroring societal inequities. Those who possess capital in society possess social and cultural capital in schools. Those who work in schools have achieved a level of social and cultural capital by virtue of making their way through the school system. In order to walk through the school doors as a professional one has to have learned to master the school system and school culture; a certain fluency has been achieved, whether you are cognizant of speaking the language of schooling or not. You know. As advocates, we must recognize that there are preferred and privileged narratives in schools. We need to focus our lens to see what is not being seen and engage the voices of those who are not being heard. Consider the following example of how a school advocate (a social worker and educational leadership graduate student) sees, hears, and is not silent about what she sees and hears:

> I walk into the office and I see all these black and brown children.
> And they are children even though they are in middle school.
> And I think they are missing class . . . they are missing their education.
> And I ask one boy, "So why are you here?"
> And he says, "I don't know."
> And I say, "What do you mean you don't know? What happened in your classroom?"
> And he says, "I don't know. I was working with my friend and then the teacher said 'go, just go to the office!' and I went."

This advocate first works with the students in the office, and then with the administrator and the teachers to get the students back in class. Afterwards, she accesses the school database to track attendance, by period, of African-American and Latino students. The advocate and the principal decide to share the data with teachers during a staff meeting. The resulting conversations generate further questions, concerns, a commitment to addressing the loss of learning time, and a desire to hear more about what students have to say. Listening and working to transform the student narrative sparks a difficult, but critical, participatory inquiry process at the site.

Understanding Narratives Define a School Community

Sterling's (2001) statement, "Words have power" (p. 14), could be reframed as language has power because language consists of more than mere words. Speaking the right language or dialect can open or close opportunity to enter different cultures and form respectful relationships. People exist in language environments. Language is foreign to the person who does not speak it, but not to the native who was born into it and sees his or her world from inside that language. Being able to speak different languages enables one to enter into the cultural space of those who speak the language. It is a gift to speak any language. The world gets described in certain ways by the language being spoken and by the group's language. The same holds for dialects, and even professional or craft languages that enable individuals to talk about what they do within various fields of practice. Wootton (2015) shares how science evolved with the acceptance and use of new words that helped to define and extend both the language and possibilities for scientific understanding. Teachers talk to teachers and educators use language in certain ways. Medical doctors do the same, as do landscape architects, gardeners, chefs, etc. Students and peers have their own language, too. Language gets introduced and changes how we define ourselves.

Carl Anthony (1995) shares the story about how the poor Irish working next to the Black slaves were united in their distain for the oppressive conditions of their lives; until those in power started talking to the Irish about how they were different from the Blacks because they were White. Thus, the linguistic shift to Whiteness gave the term and person greater power and privilege. Another example comes from the invention of the term Hispanic. Up until the 1970s the census considered Mexicans, Cubans, and Puerto Ricans White. Then in 1970, the term Hispanic was created; the groups that were distinct but contained in the White census category were renamed by the census as a singular and separate Hispanic group (Bishop & Vargas, 2015). Thus, Hispanic was born from the desire to identify a separate group of people. Ironically, just as "White" fails to capture the distinct differences between Germans and Greeks, "Hispanic" fails to capture the distinct differences between Mexicans and Cubans. In the same vein, people with European or Middle Eastern ancestry are White in the United States. Conversations about race are made more difficult because our language, our thoughtless words, toss us into broad categories where we lose parts of the stories emerging from our ancestral ethnic groups and our family stories. Some European-Americans conflate "American" with Whiteness; or minimize rich and necessary cultural differences by saying we are all Americans. To escape the generalized "American" positioning, racial identity gets hyphenated in order to celebrate and connect to ones roots with terms such as African-American, Mexican-American, European-American, etc. Educators are encouraged to help all students explore and discover what is best in their racial and ethnic identity. Such words mean something.

Humans live in language ecosystems where language flows in numerous ways, and stops only at those points where the language is not understood, no longer spoken, or is silenced by those who hold some languages as the dominate community language, superior to other languages; the language "I" speak and understand; the language "I" expect you to speak and understand, etc.

The families, schools, communities, and cultures can be described as language and narrative ecosystems. People live in language and narrative systems. Language and learning are bound together and are linked to the sense we make of the world (Briscoe, Arriaza, & Henze, 2009; Britton, 1970; Bruner, 1986, 1990, 1996, 2002; Smith, 1975, 2006). Family stories are more self-contained, but still leak out into the neighborhood and beyond. Families have stories inside and outside of the self-contained unit. School narratives are generally set in neighborhoods and communities, and are frequently used as evidence about the neighborhood or community's success or failure.

Some languages, stories, and ways of describing families, schools, communities, and cultures become powerful and expansive. That is why it is important to look at and listen to the language and stories in any community. In the broadest sense, there are approximately 6800–6900 distinct languages in the world today. As trade languages such as English expand, vast numbers of regional and tribal languages become threatened with extinction (McWhorter, 2001). The numerous languages of the Native-American peoples have been reduced due to human and cultural genocide. There was a historical and political process where European settlers moved into the lands populated by Indigenous people, who were subsequently killed by disease and murder or pushed out of prime real estate by European guns, germs, and steel (Diamond, 1999). Native-American languages and cultures were supplanted by English and "American" culture. Thankfully, there is an active effort by Native-Americans and their allies to retain what remains of those cultures and to renew languages and cultures that have been marginalized by European-American expansion. The point in sharing this information is to look at and affirm what has been lost whenever one way of being reduces or eliminates another way of being. It is important to see, by opening our eyes to a history where collective denial has enabled European-Americans not to see or even look, and to recognize that very little has been done to take responsibility for the destruction of the cultures whose land was taken by disease, murder, and treachery. This perspective empathizes with the loss of the Native-American and other cultures and languages; it is an attempt to reframe how to view the fact that languages and stories that sustained numerous cultures are disappearing from the planet, just like so many plants and animals. Cultural diversity has value. Added to the empathy and sense of loss for what is gone is the recognition that different languages and different stories describe the world in numerous ways that have also been lost for the most part. As advocates, we appreciate that those who speak more than one language have the capacity to understand more fully what it means to see and hear the world described in different ways and with different narratives.

Student advocates understand the value of different dialects (Smith, 1975). The African-American, Black, or Ebonics dialect is a language that designates an African-American experience within a community. In other words, the Black dialect has value to those in the culture from which it emerges. It is vital to honor and respect the Black dialect as a cultural expression, and as a language with its own unique grammar and linguistic structure. It is important to invite African-American youth to learn a standard English dialect, not because the standard dialect is better, but because the standard dialect is the language spoken by the dominant population in businesses and schools outside and beyond the neighborhoods and communities where Black youth frequently live. Advocates must open themselves to understanding the variety of local dialects in order to interact in a respectful manner and make positive cultural connections.

It is important to know the cultural history within any language.

Reflective Moment 3.1

Please take the time to write your responses to the questions in order to define your own thinking about language in your community. Again, consider the perspective taken in this text. Consider the implications of your responses for the students you serve.

Developing a greater language and cultural connection to the community where you are working or with any child you are trying to help and understand, it is important to ask:

- What is the primary language spoken at home?
- What is the primary language spoken with friends?
- What is the primary language of the classroom?
- How many different languages and dialects are spoken at school?
  - Who speaks what language or dialect?
  - Is the language respected? Marginalized?
- How can mutual respect be nurtured within the dialect or between those speaking the dialect and others?
- How can I honor the different languages and dialects spoken at school?

People use language to make sense of the world where they find themselves. People are born into languages that predate their existence in the country, region, or family of their origin. They learn the language of the era and time they were born into; for instance, no child picks up Elizabethan English unless that is the language their parents and community speak. Languages emerge and evolve in communities. Language is alive and continually grows in new directions, describing the world afresh and clarifying what has been fuzzy, vague, or lost in some gap that has not been described with words. Over time, words take on different meanings and nuance. New words emerge, and unused words are lost, such as the slang term "groovy" from the 1960s and 1970s. There is a language ecology that helps us to understand and appreciate the flow and evolution of the words we use to describe the world.

Toward Nurturing Narrative Ecosystems that Promote Learning

There are narrative ecosystems, too. There is never one story. Every story has infinite alternative stories. Thus there are vast networks of stories told and stories that are possible in the narrative ecosystems where humans find themselves. The aliveness of and gaps in language cannot be over-emphasized, nor can the understanding that all stories have gaps, different possibilities for interpretation, and openings for new or alternative understandings (Boyd, 2009; Briscoe et al., 2009; Bruner, 2002; Gergen, 2009; Goleman et al., 2012; Lakoff & Johnson, 1999; Mehl-Madrona, 2010; Monk et al., 1997; Peavy, 2004; Taylor, 2007).

Stories are told about individuals, families, schools, communities, states, nations, etc. Stories are told from the first, second, and third person perspective. Writers working on professional publications are told not to use the first person to avoid taking a personal, editorial, or grandstanding position in the text. Interpersonally, we tell stories about ourselves. In families, groups, and communities, we tell stories about others. Others tell stories about us and about themselves. Our minds are likened to being story processors and our lives as narratives, which are essentially "post hoc fabrications" (Haidt, 2012, p. 282). We tell ourselves about our capacity to learn and we tell stories about how vibrant or dull our school or school day was. Yet, our stories and life narratives are open to continuous deletion, expansion, and revision. Not summarizing our life narratives on paper (which always leaves something out), capturing something on film, or trying to walk away from them will save them from change via reinterpretation. In other words, people are continuously composing and changing their stories. While some personal and social stories are more stable than others, all stories are open to new perspectives and new openings for seeing, hearing, and acting.

Almost every story and ethical enactment has elements such as plot, character, perspective or point of view, theme, setting, and usually conflict or challenge. When analyzing stories, the critic will look at the story elements. When composing stories, authors move the reader along by describing story elements in a way that places the reader into the narrator's story world. It's crucial to understand that there can be conflicting narratives, where administrators and school publications tell one story and talk in the teachers' lounge offers very different stories. When working in a school, it is important to search for the differing narratives in order to develop positive, learning, and life-enhancing stories and counter-narratives. The crucial point is that there are numerous storytellers and multiple stories in any group or organization. The role of the advocate is to actively listen before taking a role in constructing positive, learning, and life-enhancing stories that focus on the success of students, families, teachers, and administrators.

Gossip and Shaming. As advocates enter conversations at school to find out about the school stories, it is important to recognize that gossip seeps into many individual, group, and collective stories and impacts school organizations (Beaudoin & Taylor, 2004; Boyd, 2009). Gossip can influence community norms and even control others socially. Those recruited into gossip are invited to join select and usually covert cliques who offer or repeat information that might not be public, and for that matter, accurate. In schools, gossip can be about administrators, teachers, counselors, school psychologists, special educators, parents, students, and just about anybody. Gossip is negative and toxic in organizations because it infects the entire community discourse with misinformation and provides those engaged in gossip with status and power that is contrary to enhancing overall community life and wellness. Gossip is linked to bullying and controlling others in ways that oppress and limit them as people and learners.

Shaming is also a powerful way to hold individuals in place or to prevent them from expressing themselves. Shaming is frequently projected upon middle-school girls, but such practices can be found among boys and girls, as well as men and women. Shaming sustains rather than breaks sexist stereotypes: "Did you see what she wore?" Or "He can't hit the ball." Shaming can enter into the discourse and become integrated in ways of gossiping about others.

Thus, in listening to stories generated inside and outside of school, it is vital not to judge or put down, but to actively wonder about the most positive, learning, and life-enhancing stories individuals and groups can generate (Lewis et al., 2010) for future forming. We must listen for less-than-pleasant details, narratives educators may not wish to hear, if we wish to collaboratively create alternative, healthier resolutions. Remember, listening takes time. There is never enough time to hear all the possible stories that fill any school. Thus, it is important to realize that there are alternative and untold stories to every story listened to and embraced. There are also always story gaps where additional details might offer new insights, understandings, and possibilities for new decisions, goals, and pathways for action, too. There are also ways to influence community stories and individual stories, which will be explored in the subsequent chapters.

NOW: The Composing Moment and the Story Told

The empty page leaves the writer with many decisions, which is a process of moving from possibility to closure. Stories are shaped by specific life contexts, situations, themes, etc. Thus, the composing moment is much more open, whereas with the story told there is closure that is left open to interpretation by the gaps left in the story being told. There are always multiple ways to see a story and there are always gaps where certain pieces of the story have not been told (Lawson, 2001; Monk et al., 1997). Hence, there is openness in composing a new story and openness in interpreting an existing story about our own learning or school experience.

On one hand, even when the author is staring at a blank page or the speaker is preparing to share an unprepared story, composing what is written or said is in the moment; there is a presence to the activity, even if that activity is daydreaming and ruminating about not coming up with ideas. On the other hand, existing stories have enough substance to be heard or read. Those listening should be curious about what something means or what has been left out, but the story has enough substance to exist, post hoc, told after the fact. With existing stories the life world gets explained, the mind/brain of the characters is considered, and moment-to-moment thoughts are searched and even explicitly explored in some way. At most, the everyday school stories that are told can be revised and told from a new or different perspective. In the everyday school stories being composed, the life world depends on context, the mind/brain is open, and moment-to-moment thought is just that—occurring in the moment and passing away to another thought. The composing process is filled with endless possibilities. There are possibilities for new school story directions and interpretations within stories that have been told. The point here is that there is much more freedom and possibility in composing new school stories, which might say something about mobility in the United States and the importance of inviting new kids in school to explore positive ways of being.

People's lives are made up from both stories that are told and stories being composed in their heads each and every moment of their lives. In the United States and other consumerist cultures, people often define themselves by what they have and strive desperately to get more products and goods (Kasser & Kanner, 2004; Schor, 1998). Some argue that the mindless consumerism is not only harmful psychologically and socially, but actually is creating a culture of extinction that shows little respect for the living planet (Bender, 2003). For advocates, it is crucial to consider the school or learning story told and being composed in the moment, always asking and wondering about helping each child fully understand that to be human is to be continuously learning and storying regardless of what props and things you might have.

Assessment via Stories

People are assessed socially through the stories they tell and by the stories told about them (Boyd, 2009). By the same token, schools, organizations, and communities are assessed by the stories they tell and by the stories that are told about them. Listening to stories without judgment and not making conclusions about the stories told and being told is crucial to advocates. This is especially true with learning stories, including individual, group, and community learning stories. In the meantime, it is important to develop story pathways for creating, reinterpreting, or celebrating the learning stories at schools. Such action requires participatory leadership.

Reflective Moment 3.2

Please take the time to write your responses to the questions in order to define your own thinking about the questions and the perspective being raised in this text. Consider the implications of your responses for the students you serve.

Advocates are wise to explore the personal narratives of those they work with:

- How do individuals see themselves as learners?
- How do students describe their experiences of school?
- How do families describe their experiences at your school site?
- How do specific groups see school?
- How does the community see the school and the students in the school?

Fostering a New Narrative: From Comorbidity to Covitality

Michael Furlong and his colleagues are at the beginning stages of moving the youth development conversation from a deficit-focused discussion of comorbidity to one that explores ways to enhance covitality. "The term covitality encompasses youths' capacity for living a life with meaning and purpose" (Furlong et al., 2013, p. 4). Although in the early stages, their robust research agenda and efforts have resulted in the development of the Social Emotional Health Survey (SEHS), a broad measure that assesses multiple psychological constructs that are empirically supported as contributing to the mental health of youth (Dowdy et al., 2015; Furlong et al., 2013; You, Furlong, Felix, & O'Malley, 2015). Building on the positive youth development literature, Furlong and his associates were interested in moving comorbidity's concentration on the co-occurrence of multiple disease states toward looking at the co-occurrence of multiple positive psychological traits, which was defined as covitality. In other words, Furlong and his associates are working to re-story how professionals talk about youth development by moving from a deficit-focused story to a strengths-based narrative which asserts that youth have the capacity to live their lives with meaning and purpose. A vital part of their research has pointed to the importance of fostering as many positive psychological dispositions and traits as possible because "the combination of strengths matters more than the individual components—the sum is greater than the parts" (Furlong et al., 2013, p. 4). Help students cultivate the greatest combination of strengths possible.

The specific factors that define the covitality construct will be explored later. The important point here is that there are measures being developed that can help student advocates, especially school psychologists, transform the stories about relational wellness and learning power for individual students and for school communities. Furlong and his associates are making important contributions to changing the ways leaders and the public story the lives of students.

Storying Participatory Leadership in Action

Participatory leaders accept the responsibility and recognize that "interpretations of the world are multivocal" (Bruner, 1996, p. 15). There are many voices in every community. Like all citizens, participatory leaders recognize that professionals participate in communities to construct a world via conversations and actions. Truth is not merely given by someone claiming to hold it; truth is a participatory construction and is fostered best in schools where methodologies assess what works to help all youth fulfill their potential in specific communities and contexts (Lewis & Borunda, 2006). Thus, it is important to define methodologies for building pathways that seek truth or successful working in action. Random action results in random outcomes. Mindful action is more likely to result in goals that can be assessed, adjusted, and achieved. Participatory leadership builds upon mindful action by advocating for nurturing relationships with individuals, groups, and other community members that build pathways to defining goals that can be assessed, adjusted, and achieved.

Chapter Summary

Learning power in schools is enhanced by open inquiry into what works in local school settings, interrogating existing privileged narratives, recognizing how narratives define schools, and constructing narratives that promote vibrant and inclusive learning communities. Constructing such narratives is dependent upon recognizing that the composing moment is now, not at some later point. In order to move in the moment, it is crucial to assess current narratives and stories operating in the school, and to offer pathways into more life-enhancing learning narratives, such as that offered by the covitality construct being developed by Michael Furlong and his colleagues.

The chapter presents participatory leadership as a form of storying that is employed by advocates to build upon mindful actions and nurturing relationships with individuals, groups, and other stakeholders that build pathways to defining goals that can be assessed, adjusted, and achieved.

4 The Participatory Inquiry Process (PIP)

Participatory truth is species-specific, culture-bound, and evolving. It is not absolute, but it is not subjective. It is inter-subjective within the culture, within the accepted discourse.

(Henryk Skolimowski, 1994, p. xix)

This chapter gives an overview of the participatory inquiry process (PIP); the specific PIP phases are described in Chapters 6–9. Before detailing PIP, it is important to consider ethics, which are central to informed decisions directed toward ends that have relational, aspirational, and life-affirming consequences in schools. We are speaking of ethics in the broad sense of the term, which are tied to both personal and professional decisions, actions, and the recognition that "an ethical expert is nothing more or less than a full participant in a community" (Varela, 1992, p. 24). Life-affirming, solar ethics are those aspirational ethics that inform a way of living; a form of loving life by pouring our hearts into living, deciding, and acting as compassionately and passionately as possible; in other words, putting on a good show and doing the best we can, regardless of our own weakness and flaws, in any given circumstances we face (Cupitt, 1995).

There are plenty of decisions and actions available to those working in schools, and sadly, every year many schools adopt new and expensive programs designed to provide tidy answers to the numerous educational challenges facing their community. At the same time, the educational vendors usually lack significant understanding, knowledge, appreciation, or commitment to the local community being helped. Vendors exist for profit, making money to bring about some usually short-term change, and leaving the community when the money is gone. There are parades of highly paid vendors and educational consultants who take part in this corporate educational circus. This text is about helping those with or interested in understanding, knowing, appreciating, and making a commitment to help public schools and communities educate citizens who have a sense of their own learning power and the skills to promote the well-being of themselves, their families, their fellow citizens, and the land to which they belong. Communities need local and engaged ethical professional practitioners interested in helping all students live up to their greatest potential. School communities need people with an aspirational ethic who can join with others to lifescape their schools in ways that bring about sustainable local development measured by students' learning power and well-being. There is not a magic bullet; there is a continuous and ongoing process that never ends because people and communities have the potential to continually develop as long as they are alive. Organizations have a responsibility to be living attempts to engage participants, and communities have a responsibility to be gardens that cultivate competent citizens, not colonies where the latest corporate fad sucks resources and energy from the community. Action research calls for inviting students to participate in the research process. In fact, Youth Participatory Action Research (YPAR) can be integrated into PIP by researchers who invite youth to become co-researchers in lifescaping their schools.

Schools should be pillars of democracy and, while it is important to recognize that STEM (Science, Technology, Engineering, Math) programs are critical in our society, it is also vital to recognize music, drama, art, industrial arts, and all the other areas where youth can develop a sense of competence. The movement to revise STEM to STEAM (Science, Technology, Engineering, Art, Math) is in the right direction, but it is necessary to put resources into music, drama, art, and industrial arts. Reflecting as parents, we made sure our own children were grounded in math and science. Rolla has one child who majored in Marine Biology and became a nurse program after volunteering two years in the Peace Corps in Mozambique where she recognized the need for competent health care professionals; Rolla's other child majored in Geology and Physics and is currently pursuing a graduate degree in Environmental Engineering. Peg's oldest child, who majored in Human Biology while earning a Master's in Modern Thought and Literature, is currently working at a housing project health clinic and will be entering medical school. Her second child chose an interdisciplinary Urban Studies major and has spent two summers working with inner-city youth on a Murals and Arts Program as the resident lyricist instructor. Her third child is entering a public high school that offers multiple pathways including an IB program. Our kids were grounded in math and science, but they were also encouraged to pursue the arts, music, drama, dance, sport, cooking and other life-enhancing endeavors. Our point in sharing these personal stories is to frame all efforts to improve schools for all students as both personal and professional. We hope all students have the opportunity to cultivate their learning power as our kids have. Schools have an obligation to engage kids in the understanding that to be human is to be learning throughout life. That is a solar ethical stance that will be explored more fully below.

Ethical Action as Mapping the World We Want to Construct

Seeing, hearing, and speaking out is crucial, and connected to ethical action and how we map choices in living life, both personally and professionally. Ethics and morals have similar roots. The word ethics is derived from the Greek "ethos" just as the word moral was derived from the Roman or Latin term "mores." Ethos referred to the accepted ways of doing things within Greek society, just as mores referred to the ways of ancient Rome. They are not synonymous today. Ethics are tied more closely to the philosophy of morality, whereas morals refer more closely to the accepted standards of a person, group, or society. For the purposes of this book, ethics refers to actions guided by standards and aspirational values influencing human conduct and relationships between individuals, within groups and professions, between groups, as members of the human community, and as part of the web of life. To take a simple second-grade binary ethical perspective: are you nice (respectful) or are you mean (not respectful) toward other people, animals, and things? As we mature, we grow up and think more deeply about our ethical actions as professionals, family members, and citizens. We define aspirational ethics that call us to do the "right thing," "just thing," "compassionate thing," etc.

The vastness of ethics and ethical action must be affirmed. Otherwise, it is far too easy for individuals to hide from living into their responsibility as active members of a world community where we are all life citizens within local biological and social ecosystems and niches (e.g., Bowers, 1997; Capra, 2002; Goleman et al., 2012; Leopold, 1949; Naess, 1988, 2002; Nash, 1989; Peavy, 2004; Schumacher, 1973; Sessions, 1995; Smith & Williams, 1999; Sterling, 2001; Williams & Brown, 2012). Ethics are guidelines created by people for mapping out how to make the best possible decisions in a wide array of circumstances. Yet, ethics has evolved dramatically in human history. In the past, it was ethical to enslave, to kill members of rival tribes or nations, to hold women as lesser humans, to destroy vast forest ecosystems, to use beautiful religious or cultural landmarks for target practice, etc. Few people in the United States would argue that slavery is a way of life that should be preserved or that women should be treated as chattel; collectively we know slavery and the oppression of women are wrong. Just as we know burning witches is wrong. Such overt positions are reprehensible by today's ethical standards, and even seem odd to talk about, although they were considered ethical practices and enactments in the past, even in what is now the United States, land of the free. Consider Thomas Jefferson, the slave-owning founding father who wrote "all men [sic] are created equal" into the Declaration of Independence. Jefferson had the idea of equality, though flawed, but in practice his slaves were mere property and exploited to the degree it was profitable. During the subsequent years, we citizens of the United States have struggled to take Jefferson's notion of equality in a more inclusive direction; freeing slaves after the Civil War, granting women the right to vote in the early twentieth century, fighting for civil rights in the 1960s, and recognizing homosexuals as people in the early years of the twenty-first century. Jefferson was greatly flawed, but the aspirational ethic driving the people of the United States took what was good with his idea of equality and moved it to include all people.

The point is that equality, freedom, and dignity are concepts that evolve in relation to the aspirational ethics guiding our practices. Ethical acts have expanded over the years, even though our sense of right does not always align. Witness various forms of covert and micro-aggressions that take place in conversations, such as when a European-American teacher tells an African-American student who is doing well in class that she is a credit to her race. The teacher may mean well, but the message is an unconscious micro-aggression that implies something negative about African-Americans. Thankfully, people can and do learn and our sense of right evolves over time because our national discourse seems to have aspirational ethics woven to some degree into it.

Haidt (2012) shows that our sense of what is right changes and evolves over time, but our sense of what is right divides people into various groups that judge what is right from differing perspectives. At the very least, what is right is not written in stone; our consensus of what is right changes over time, and thankfully in the United States, what is right seems to evolve toward greater compassion toward differences and the affirmation that we are citizens of a life-community. Ethical action is complex and lends itself to multiple and evolving interpretations that cannot be limited to interactions between people and human systems but extended to include the relationship between personal and planetary wellness and health.

Ethics is a subcategory within the study of philosophy, and it is important to note that philosophy has impacted psychology and the helping professions much more profoundly than most academics and practitioners acknowledge in their quest for the most current, cutting edge theory (Alexander & Shelton, 2014). There are arguments against ethics (Caputo, 1993), ethics as obligation (Williams, 1985), ethics of identity (Appiah, 2005), situation ethics (Fletcher, 1966), flow of life (Gilbert, 2009), a land ethic (Leopold, 1949; Nash, 1989), and more. Ethics stretches to define relationships between and among similar and diverse people, as well as with the land community to which we all belong. Bowers (1997, 2000, 2001, 2003) warns that connecting culture, environment, ethics, and education is vital to creating an ecologically sustainable future. Understanding the scope of ethics helps to put the complexity and roots of professional ethics into the study of how people should treat each other as well as the rest of the world they find themselves part of. The essential point here is that the study of ethics is a lifelong endeavor and not an activity one merely checks off as having completed as part of an educational program or professional development workshop. Another point is that ethical action moves beyond consideration of what is right between and among people and human systems and toward a deeper aspirational ethical understanding of the human relationship to the life systems where they exist as planetary citizens and participants in community narratives. As Kearney (2002) says, "If we possess narrative sympathy—enabling us to see the world from the other's point of view—we cannot kill. If we do not, we cannot love" (p. 140). To be true to ethics as a continuous evolving process is to be constantly reflecting upon one's actions and the consequences of those actions. Even guided by aspirational ethics, it is vital to note the need to be humble and embrace an "ethics without absolutes" because "life is a complex adaptive network in which everything is codependent and coevolves . . . [meaning] absolutism must give way to relationalism" (Taylor, 2007, p. 355). As mentioned earlier, schools are theaters where student advocates relate to their community and take ethical action to promote well-being and learning power for all students. Please bear this in mind as you move forward in your professional development.

Simply put, professional ethics are guidelines to help guide professional actions, but all ethical action should be put in a context of one's citizenship in local, regional, national, cultural, and world communities. Be humble. Be concrete and embodied in the context where you find yourself. Still, take time to review your profession's ethical standards. (The ethical standards for school counselors and school psychologists are available online; see: www.schoolcounselor.org/files/EthicalStandards2010.pdf; and www.nasponline.org/standards/professionalcond.pdf; and www.aamft.org/imis15/content/legal_ethics/code_of_ethics.aspx. And the standards for administrators can be found at www.ctc.ca.gov/educator-prep/standards/CPSEL-booklet-2014.pdf.)

Ethical action is central to professional practice, and shaping one's ethical stance is a lifelong endeavor regardless of your profession because, at their best, ethics can inform actions and press individuals and supportive groups of individuals to wonder about and question the ideology guiding the dominant culture. This is true of schools, too, where the ideologies and practices are frequently taken for granted and unexplored. We must begin inquiring into life how we live it (Newbury, 2014). Ideology is a comprehensive view, a worldview that shapes the way people look at the world they are part of and accept as the "way things are" or as "what is real," "true," etc. Ideology undergirds the hidden curriculum and our taken-for-granted ways of seeing and being in the world. A considered ideology can be used to shape how professionals view data and respond to challenges.

The data showing that African-American youth are the least represented group in universities and colleges may be viewed in differing ways, according to ideology. One group could say that the data show African-American youth are not interested in school, not as intelligent, or other rot that justifies the current situation. Another group could say that the

---

Reflective Moment 4.1

Please take the time to write your responses to the questions in order to define your own thinking about the questions and the perspective being raised in this text. Consider the ethical implications of your responses for the students you serve.

- Name two things that come to mind as you review the professional ethical standards for your specialization.
- Please comment on what your ethical standards say about things you see at your site.
- Please comment on what your ethical standards say about things you hear at your site.
- Please comment on what your ethical standards say about what ethical actions you should take regarding what you see and hear.

---

data reveal that there continue to be opportunity gaps that prevent African-American youth from attaining their potential. One position shows a lack of faith in the learning power of all kids, and the other position shows a fundamental faith in the learning power of all kids. Obviously, the argument is simplistic but the point is that ethical practice forces professionals to unpack ideology and unexamined assumptions about current conditions. The challenge is getting up close enough to the kids to find out how to experience and see school and to figure out solutions with them to help them realize their potential as learners and as citizens.

Educators and counselors swim in cultural waters alive with mores, ethos, and ideologies. We must be prepared to unpack and understand ethical relationships, as well as define those that will help guide us in our professional practice, and for that matter, our decision making in the world where diverse "other" people and the entire biosphere are impacted by how humans relate to each other and to the sacred living systems where they dwell (Skolimowski, 1993). Knowing about ethical relationships and ecological integrity requires that theories that guide action be met with skeptical empiricism, continually tested and re-tested in the context where the theories are implemented. More importantly for this text, knowing about ethical relationships and ecological integrity presses us to use tools such as action research and appreciative inquiry to lifescape the communities where we want to dwell. Action research and appreciative inquiry enable us to question ourselves and to recognize and confront institutionalized oppression and privilege; action research and appreciative inquiry empowers us to live a solar ethic, burning brightly like the sun, as responsible agents in professions and cultures capable of defining and redefining their evolving ethics in order to enhance our individual and collective experience of life, as well as the ecological integrity and vitality of the planet.

Ethics and Truth: Action Research in Local Settings

Action and truth become connected to what works successfully to bring about effective results (Hansen, 2006b, 2007; Hayes et al., 1993; Mead, 1932/2002; Peirce, 1923/1998; Pepper, 1942). The four phases and nine steps in PIP emerge from active and engaged forms of promoting change and accountability, such as participatory action research and appreciative inquiry (e.g. Cooperrider & Whitney, 2005; Heron & Reason, 1997; Reason & Bradbury, 2008; Reason & Hawkins, 1988; Rowell, 2005, 2006; Torbert, 2004; Whiston, 1996). Action research in this text is defined as a PIP that engages members of the school community in conversations, reflection, analysis, and action directed to enhance student, faculty, administrator, family, and other community members' well-being and learning power. The inquiry process does not foreground such things as standardized high stakes exams; students' personal/social competence, decision making skills, personal learning power, and sense of purpose come first. Student projects, portfolios, and demonstrated competence are more important than scores on standardized tests. The inquiry process always tries to take into account the lives students actually live and the obstacles they define as blocking their dignity, well-being, and learning (Newbury, 2014).

Advocates for Change

Ethics and action research are tied together in promoting principles of social justice and democratic practice (Brydon-Miller, 2008). PIP grows out from the action research tradition, and attempts to invite diverse community members in schools to become active advocates for change, looking, listening, and responding to what they see and hear in order to promote the well-being and learning power of all persons within specific school communities. The crucial point here is that the individual researcher is but one member of the local community in a process where human relationships are key to transformative change (Gergen & Gergen, 2008). In fact, "Action researchers must remain mindful of the complex nature of balancing individual and collective action and the relationships of power and privilege which inevitably frame these processes of decision making" (Gergen & Gergen, 2008, p. 202). As described in this text, developing deep relational connections within the setting and context where the practitioner–researcher finds him or herself is vital to promoting dialogues about possibilities and actions to be taken in the specific school setting. Action research is a "practical art" that invites transformative dialogue about taking action to "realize visions of what the world can become" (Gergen & Gergen, 2008, p. 167).

Action research has a long history in teacher education promoting educational reform (e.g., Adelman, 1993; Somekh & Zeichner, 2009). Dana's (2013) work provides very accessible action research for teachers and even administrators, but school counselors and school psychologists are not central to her work; this text is meant to provide a pathway for school counselors, school psychologists, school social workers, and other youth advocates to join with administrators, teachers, and other school community members. School advocates bring essential knowledge, context, and individual contacts to the examination of school practices. These helping professionals have access and relationships with students and families from historically under-served populations. From a community perspective, school counselors, school psychologists, school social workers, and other educational advocates are uniquely positioned to engage students and community members who are not thriving in the current system(s).

The educational goal of this current work is guided by an understanding Reason and Bradbury (2001, p. 2) offered:

> A primary purpose of action research is to produce practical knowledge that is useful to people in the everyday conduct of their lives. A wider purpose of action research is to contribute through this practical knowledge to the increased well-being ... of human persons and communities, and to a more equitable and sustainable relationship with the wider ecology of the planet of which we are an intrinsic part.

We would add to this, as educator advocates, the primary purpose of action research is to lifescape school communities using practical, local knowledge that is useful to the professionals, stakeholders, and community interested in promoting the well-being and learning power of all students. Indeed, we stand with other educators who work to include students and their voices in the process of transforming schools to reflect community values and understandings (Gillen, 2014; Harris et al., 2014).

PIP is a lifescaping process that involves engaged action-oriented interventions in local communities that are assessed and evolve via continuous feedback and dialogue; the methodology does not necessarily include rigorous empirical outcome research using randomized experimental and control groups. The action-oriented goals formulated in the PIP process generate local knowledge about what works best in the school and with the students where the practitioner is working. PIP does not mean ignoring outcome research, it means engaging in a continuous change and accountability process directed toward building the most life-enhancing learning community possible. PIP does not diminish the importance of outcome research, but it does assert that practitioners have a professional obligation to get to know and work with the communities they serve and to continually work to find and assess the best ways to inspire all kids to cultivate their learning power and sense of well-being. PIP is about future forming and lifescaping, not about describing the way things are and letting them be as they are.

PIP is an approach that enables helping professionals to take mindful steps toward carefully negotiated goals that address problems and challenges facing school learning communities. PIP enables professionals interested in school transformation to utilize a tool that can inform and guide the change process toward aspirational ethics and goals embraced by the community. There are key and vital resources that can help school counselors take action to develop their comprehensive school counseling programs (e.g., ASCA, 2012; Dimmitt, Carey, & Hatch, 2007; Galassi & Akos, 2007; Gysbers & Henderson, 2012; Holcomb-McCoy, 2007; Johnson et al., 2006; Paisley & Hubbard, 1994; Squier et al., 2014; Stephens & Lindsey, 2011; Stone & Dahic, 2004; Young & Kaffenberger, 2009). PIP is one of the pathways that invites students and other community members to participate in the change process.

PIP is not a silver bullet, but it is a continuous process that engages professionals as participatory leaders in achieving goals focused on doing (at least) one thing better and tapping into the learning power of all students (Lewis & Borunda, 2006). Importantly, although spelled out in phases and steps, PIP is non-linear because, depending on one's social capital and understanding, there are times when the student advocate can cycle into the collaborative work at later steps and other times when they must loop back to an earlier step in the process. There are other times when advocates are directed to implement a program handed down by the district hierarchy at step seven; which means the first six steps in the process are bypassed and voices are silenced. Still, the nine steps in PIP are designed to help inform and guide student advocates' lifescaping efforts in bringing about results that can be built upon, changed, and improved in a continuous manner and in response to the feedback from the local school community where action is implemented.

Four Phases and Nine Steps in the Participatory Inquiry Process (PIP)

Phase 1: Initiating Conversations and Identifying Challenges

Step 1. Advocates must listen deeply to the content, feeling, and meaning of what is said as they begin the inquiry process by examining the school environment, accessible school data, and other school-wide sources of information that will begin to provide the school's narrative. Advocates enter the community like an anthropologist by listening to individuals and groups to hear some of the school's stories and story elements, including such characteristics as the school's strengths, assets, and perceived challenges as a learning community. Advocates try to understand the current school lifescape. Student advocates collaboratively begin to define a challenge to be addressed that could improve the school lifescape, typically a student group being under-served or marginalized. As participatory leaders, advocates facilitate the examination of challenges and aspirations. They open possibility pathways for solving a problem based on data that impacts the delivery of student services or the school as a learning community.

Step 2. Advocates facilitate conversations, dialogues, and collaborations about the school lifescape among community members including: site supervisors, professionals-in-training, school counselors, school psychologists, teachers, administrators, students, parents, and other community members. Conversations are directed toward success stories in the past, outstanding practices and traditions, possible futures, ways to transform practices, and best possible and dreamed-for student outcomes. Thought is given to deciding what data to track and identifying what challenges to address.

Phase 2: Engaged Inquiry

Step 3. Using professional resources, dialogues and engaged inquiry are initiated to explore possibilities for responses to the problem being researched. Resources within the school community are assessed and reflected on in framing how to address the challenge(s) identified and, more importantly, how to lifescape the school they want to have. Student advocates pose inquiry questions such as: What resources, services, and strategies are currently in place to serve students? What is working? What's not? What areas could be initiated, expanded, or improved?

Step 4. Using available school-based data, baseline, comparative, and data trends are investigated and reflected upon by the learning community. Additional data are collected from teachers, parents, students, and other community members. Qualitative and quantitative data are gathered through surveys, focus groups, meetings, interviews, school walk-throughs, and program observations. Student advocates support the learning com - munity in considering: What questions should be posed about the data? What do we hope to learn? What is the lifescape we want to see?

Phase 3: Collaborative Action

Step 5. Conversations about problems, challenges, and actions are directed toward defining meaningful, measurable, and realistic goals that address the challenge(s). Problems, issues, and actions are defined and shared by the learning community and a strategy(s) to address the challenge is proposed. Student advocates guide the learning community in making a choice regarding what action(s) to take in lifescaping the school community.

Step 6. Actions are taken to put the agreed upon strategy(s) into practice. Knowing the envisioned lifescape, the rationale and purpose for the action(s), student advocates can support the learning community in making adjustments based on unforeseen "glitches" in the implementation process.

Phase 4: Community Assessment and Reflection

Step 7. Student advocates assist in determining and providing venues for community assessment and reflection. Actions are reflected upon and efforts are shared, e.g., with students in the school, department members, school community, school board, college or university class, etc. Did the actions move toward the desired lifescape for the school? Results may also be used as part of a document that highlights action and practices of helping professionals in the schools, such as Flashlight PowerPoint, SPARC (Support Personnel Accountability Report Card), etc. Feedback from interested community members is reflected on and used, if possible in furthering the lifescaping efforts.

Step 8. The strategy(s) is adapted accordingly via continuing learning community reflection. Student advocates pose reflective questions such as: What would you do differently? What can we do to further lifescape this area?

Step 9. Action is taken to put the revised strategy(s) into practice, and necessary steps are repeated. Student advocates assist in setting a time frame to revisit what has been done and the strategy(s) being implemented. Like expiration dates on milk cartons, a time is set in order to revisit, reassess, revise, and renew practice.

The four phases and nine steps in PIP are presented in a linear and sequential manner that enables those following them to move in a certain order. At the same time, although a sequential heuristic, the phases and steps may loop back and some practitioners may begin at step four and loop back to step one, etc. Use the steps as a guide to addressing complex challenges in complex systems, not as a rigid set of rules or a single-minded recipe that must be adhered to in sequence in order to achieve positive results. PIP is a reflective method that is focused on continuous improvement to lifescape communities. PIP is a dialogical and reflective method of lifescaping communities. PIP is aligned with and practitioners are encouraged to use PIP in conjunction with the 4-R process described in Chapter 5.

Reflective Moment 4.2

In the case of this text, action is directed toward exploring the question: How does this professional action enhance the lives of students, the community, and the life-system to which we all belong in ways that enhance justice, beauty, or ecological integrity? To begin this work on an individual level, questions could be framed in this way:

- How are students better off because of my actions?
  - How do students experience more care and support at school because of my actions?
  - How am I helping students find pathways to meaningful participation at school?
  - How am I helping students achieve the high expectations defined in the school?

Exploring such questions is a never-ending endeavor.

Advocacy and Participatory Leadership

Reflect briefly on what you have read and done in this chapter focused on the participatory inquiry process. As a student advocate, you have an overview of PIP and can begin thinking about conducting action research to lifescape your school by addressing a problem or challenge, small or large. PIP's action research approach is not going to teach you to eat a watermelon whole; PIP is about breaking the process into four phases and nine steps that are manageable and loop back on themselves if you try to go too fast or to press the process forward beyond what your necessary allies are ready for at the moment. Chapters 6–9 will spell out the PIP phases and break them into bite-sized pieces that will enable you to engage in effective future forming at your school. The phases and steps do not proceed on their own; they are embodied by active participatory leadership, as well as what we refer to as performative focus, vital engagement, self-reflectiveness, and relational connectedness—attributes of engaged and active learners, which will be explored in the next chapter.

Advocates are wise to work closely with their other community members by introducing them to PIP, building strong relationships, sharing data, and initiating respectful dialogues directed toward lifescaping their school. In the event this dialogue is not possible with your site leader, it is important to find wise allies to help you engage in PIP as a lifescaping practice in your school. In the event you are alone, you must choose a small project within your area of responsibilities to engage in PIP; once that is done, share your work with others. The path alone is not recommended, but it is still an option in the most extreme contexts. The next chapter highlights the appreciative inquiry, the second of the two future forming practices being offered in this book.

Chapter Summary

This chapter presents the four phases and nine steps in the participatory inquiry process. The chapter begins by discussing ethics in terms of action and truth. Ethics are aspirational and practical requirements for professionals, and ultimately aspirational ethics bring out the relational nature of ourselves with others, including all living beings and the natural world. As professionals and citizens, it is important to consider ethics as a professional requirement but also as a living philosophical endeavor that informs our relationships in the world. Ethics are fundamental to informed decisions directed toward ends that have positive, life-affirming consequences in schools, and ethical action is central to professional practice, and shaping one's ethical stance can inform actions and press individuals and supportive groups of individuals to wonder about and question the ideology guiding the dominant culture. This is true of schools, where the ideologies and practices are frequently taken for granted and unexplored.

PIP grows out from the action research tradition. It has four phases and nine steps that can guide advocates for change in looking, listening, and responding to what they see and hear in order to promote the well-being and learning power of all persons within specific school communities. PIP guides practitioner efforts to lifescape the school communities where they find themselves. PIP's four phases and nine steps are expanded on in Chapters 6–9. In the next chapter, we look more deeply into appreciative inquiry's power to build on the positive core in any school.

5 Appreciative Inquiry (AI) and the 4-R Process

> Human systems grow in the direction of what they persistently ask questions about, and this propensity is strongest and most sustainable when the means and ends of inquiry are positively correlated. The single most important action a group can take to liberate the human spirit and consciously construct a better future is to make the positive core the command and explicit property of all.
>
> (Cooperrider and Whitney, 2005, p. 9)

There are different ways to take an active role in lifescaping schools. The paths used in this text emphasize the participatory inquiry process (PIP) and appreciative inquiry (AI) (Barrett & Fry, 2005; Cooperrider & Whitney, 1999, 2005; Dole, Godwin, & Moehle, 2014; Lewis et al., 2010; Preskill & Catsambas, 2006; Stavros & Torres, 2005). This chapter concentrates on appreciative inquiry (AI). Cooperrider developed the notion of appreciative inquiry in conversations with his wife, who is an artist, when she talked about how important it is for artists to have an appreciative eye when looking at works of art. Being a student of organizational development, he shifted his scholarship to studying the impact appreciative questions have upon organizations. AI orients practitioners to look for the positive core, build relationships, recognize assets, challenge underlying assumptions that take energy from cooperative capacity, and actively engage participants in creating preferred futures. AI is a future forming process, just as it is a lifescaping process.

Finding the positive core is the most crucial aspect of AI. The positive core is the central value of the organization; such as teaching all students to recognize their learning power in schools. Helping students see, hear, understand, embody, and speak out about being engaged and excited about learning would be a positive core for many schools. With AI, building relationships is about inviting individuals in organizations not to get locked into roles, but to develop connection with others in relationships that focus on enhancing the positive core. Recognizing the positive core inherent in the organization and the human assets that exist maintains focus on what is working, not what is broken; the AI orientation moves from a deficit-based or problem-focused approach toward a strengths-based stance that concentrates and builds on the positive core.

The positive core of this strengths-based stance challenges underlying assumptions and discourses, such as gossip and whining, and redirects conversations toward figuring what can be done to work together to create what is desired. AI practitioners are oriented to be affirmative, inquiry-based, and improvisational in their practice (Dole et al., 2014; Preskill & Catsambas, 2006). AI practitioners in schools:

1. *Build relationships and actively work to help individuals in school organizations connect with each other as people in learning communities rather than be locked into roles that support rigid hierarchies.* Community members including secretaries, parents, students, and custodians frequently have profound insights that should be listened to in learning communities. Such relationships do not imply that advocates have to be friends or buddies; rather, these relationships are guided by listening and mindful wonderment, rather than role or position. The relationships are artful, collaborative, and inclusive.

2. *Actively listen to each other.* AI practitioners engage in mindful wonder, which essentially means they hold back on judgment, ask curiosity questions, and actively engage in listening for what is core and most important to the person speaking. This active approach to listening also is geared toward wondering how what is being said or expressed relates to the positive core: builds relationships, recognizes assets, challenges underlying assumptions that take energy from cooperative capacity, and actively engages in future forming for the learning community. The collaborative and inclusive qualities are geared toward fostering dialogues about positive possibilities and narratives about how the system can work best to help all students learn.

3. *Align dreams in working toward the positive core and aspirations.* There are opportunities to explore dreams for a preferred future and discuss how those dreams might be aligned with enhancing the positive core of the learning community.

4. *Create a learning community where there are opportunities for people to participate and choose how to contribute.* Such thinking cannot be mandated or put into job descriptions. It is important to recognize that certain forms of contribution are by invitation and not by coercion. Encourage play and wonder.

5. *Let colleagues use their own discretion in deciding how to contribute and support those colleagues in taking both small and large action steps.* Invite. Recognize actions that are even tiny steps.

6. *Act positively about future possibilities.* This is not some attempt to have everybody wear smiley face pins or where signs are posted stating, "We are all happy." Recognizing the positive core enables each of us

to embrace the positive value of what is being done and to search for the possibilities for improving our collective practices. AI is purposefully positive without being sappy. It focuses on past successes, small and large. AI recognizes grassroots approaches as opposed to organizational hierarchies and top-down approaches, and works to help schools improve. AI invites participation and connection within learning communities. AI embraces the creative and spontaneous aspects of organizational change. In other words, being positive is focused on bringing out the best in people, and acknowledging those things and people around us who help us connect and who bring more life to our work. Being positive is using mindful wonderment to affirm past and present strengths, assets, successes, and possibilities.

AI practitioners are oriented to be positive and affirmative in their inquiries focused on positive change in schools (Willoughby & Samuels, 2009). In order to guide practice, AI embraces core principles that continue to evolve from those defined by David Cooperrider in his initial conceptualizations of AI to those who have expanded upon his work (Barrett & Fry, 2005; Dole et al., 2014; Preskill & Catsambas, 2006). The core list of eight AI principles below is adapted to align with the strengths-based eco-relational perspective:

1. *The Constructionist Principle*: Individuals and organizations exist in human and biological ecosystems. Groups of people construct their reality based on their conversations related to their human relationships and their relationships with their physical environment. Biological and social ecosystems offer many different possibilities that are reduced by relationships, decisions, and conversations that evolve and change over time. Hence, relationships and stories have a profound impact upon our reality. What we talk about shapes our actions and the reality we see.

2. *The Principle of Simultaneity*: Change and inquiry occur together. They are not separate. As soon as we ask the question, we are inviting reflection and possible change in how organizations are seen or how individuals or groups act in those organizations. Thus, inquiry is a form of intervention. Participatory inquiry is the recognition that as individuals participate in conversations they must be mindful of how inquiry leads to small and large changes in personal and organizational narratives and actions.

   Student advocates are curious and search for what works best in the district, in the school, and with the students and community where they work. Advocates employ participatory inquiry and strength-based approaches to find out what works for students, teachers, and others in their learning community.

3. *The Poetic Principle*: This is a creative and artistic expression similar to Naess' notions of "possibilism" and "relationism," where anything is possible, and that we are always in relationships with people and the physical environment where we are. In this case, organizations are like gardens and sources of endless learning, inspiration, interpretation, and action because organizations are living works in progress, and they are constantly cultivated, pruned, and changed via conversations and actions. The conversations and actions point to the creative nature of the enterprise, regardless of who the lead gardener or lifescaper is.

   Because all school programs and services being delivered are evolving works in progress, venerated positions and ready-made answers presented for acceptance *en bloc* must be drawn into question, assessed, and transformed by the participatory inquiry process or other methods concerned with successful working in one's own school and with one's students. Lifescaping efforts are always connected with the place and the people, not some pre-existing plan designed elsewhere.

4. *The Anticipatory Principle*: Our dreams, images, and imagined future pull us forward. Like hope in Pandora's box, our anticipation of a more positive future gives great meaning to what we do in our lives. In terms of educators working in schools, it is our hope that children will learn and live better lives that drives most of us forward.

5. *The Positive Principle*: If we have a positive goal or dream, we will take positive action to bring it to life. When working with others, we must offer positive affect, strong relationships, connection, and joy of achieving something special, beautiful, or meaningful together. This is where what is possible becomes more focused to the group working to bring about the life-enhancing goal.

   Education is foundational in a democratic society, and points toward diverse expression and free thought as opposed to the rigid conformity required in totalitarian regimes. Student advocates foster learning power by employing life-enhancing and health-promoting approaches that build on the human capacity to learn and desire to experience happiness in life moment-to-moment as persons and citizens. Student advocates participate as professional educators and community members in the development of a just and sustainable learning community and learning narrative that believes in the ability of all youth to make a contribution.

6. *The Wholeness Principle*: This is a key Gestalt principle, too. We are not separate from one another as people. We are not fragmented beings, divided up into numerous separate parts. As individuals, we are whole beings existing in whole social and biological ecosystems. Connectedness matters and helping all students feel connected to school is vital to helping all students live up to their greatest potential.

7. *The Ethical Enactment Principle*: This is where we walk the talk and model the change we want to be. The ethical enactment principle

is about agency, ethical action, and participatory leadership. It is not about having a big hat or big title; it is about being active and enacting mindful wonderment in the present moment. That is, actively being fully aware, listening to others with a sense of openness and curiosity about their experience and their dreamed of or ideal future. The core questions are: How am I creating the world I want to live in right now? How am I living myself in what Cupitt (1995) calls a solar ethic, where I burn brightly and creatively in every action?

Truth for student advocates has to be tested out ethically in terms of successful working in one's own school and with one's own students. Thus, truth comes to be professionally and personally developed and assessed by each advocate in his or her own school, with their own students, and in their own professional lives using sound methodologies found in science and other human fields of study.

8. *The Free Choice Principle*: Being able to choose to contribute matters. Having the agency and freedom to choose how and what we contribute is important, as is making sure that the invitation to contribute and support for contributing is always available. Choice and agency are essential, invitation is vital, and responsibility is inherent in the free choice principle.

Student advocates must find and accept the responsibility for their own voice and rigorously test the success of their own program and services by concentrating on strengths in students and the community. Developing a professional voice involves attention to practice, creativity, and mindful assessment that concentrates on building upon what is working. Student advocates act mindfully to guide all students to recognize their learning power and potential as citizens in a democratic society. Responsibility entails advocating for and protecting diverse youth, while helping them live up to their greatest potential.

Reflective Moment 5.1

This AI Interview Protocol is for graduate students but it may be adapted to suit professional development or other settings.

Appreciative Inquiry Interview Protocol

1. Think of a time in your entire experience in school communities when you felt most excited, most engaged, and most alive. What were the forces and factors that made it a great experience? What was it about you, others, and your professional program that made it a peak experience for you?

2. What do you value most about yourself, your education, and your work in the school community?
3. What are your school community's best practices (the ways it manages, its approaches, its traditions)?
4. What are the unique aspects of your work in the school community that most positively affect the spirit, vitality, and effectiveness of your program and its work educating professionals?
5. What is the core factor that "gives life" in your school community?
6. What are the three most important hopes you have to heighten the health and vitality of your school community in the future?

Based on: Ludema et al. (2000).

The 4-R Appreciate Inquiry Process: Promoting Relational Wellness

The eight AI principles as adapted are essentially a strengths-based eco-relational orientation to systems change and interventions in schools. The challenge for practitioners is not merely to read the content but to genuinely integrate the perspective into day-to-day practice. The eight principles are no silver bullet or magic pill. They simply keep advocates focused on their mission of enhancing the lives and well-being of the individuals, groups, families, and schools they serve. The principles stand as an attempt to foster mindful wonderment and life-enhancing possibilities for ourselves and for those we work with in the schools where we find ourselves.

The 4-R process used in this text integrates the appreciative inquiry 4-D process and 4-I process in a manner that can be aligned with the nine steps of PIP. The 4-D process and the four phases of AI defined by Cooperrider, Whitney, & Stavros (2003) are Discovery, Dream, Design, and Destiny. The 4-I process and the four phases of AI defined by Preskill & Catsambas (2006) are Inquire, Imagine, Innovate, and Implement. The 4-R appreciative inquiry process described in this text integrates Prilleltensky and Prilleltensky's (2006) synergy of well-being and Furlong's covitality construct into an inquiry process focused on bringing about relational wellness measured by results that emerge from actions directed toward personal, organizational, and school community change (see Figure 5.1).

Relational wellness can be defined as relationships and interactions grounded in mutual respect and the shared goal of promoting the learning power of individuals, groups, and the organization; relational wellness described in this text is linked with the notion that covitality is enhanced by fostering multiple positive psychological traits (Furlong et al., 2013).

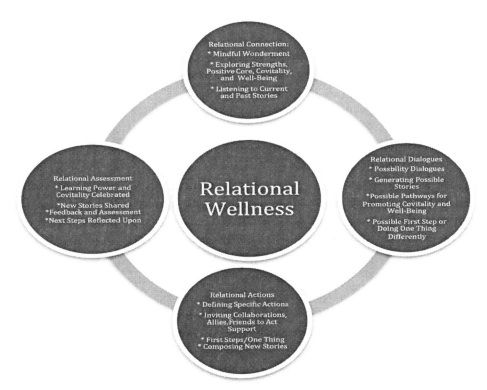

Figure 5.1 The 4-R Process.

Relational wellness is linked to promoting learning power, which is the capacity of individuals, groups, and the organization to define and strive to reach specific goals, competencies, and high expectations; learning power is also having the resilience to adjust goals, get help, and expend effort in achieving personal or group competence, high expectations, and potential. Relational wellness includes general well-being, which is a state of cognitive, emotional, spiritual happiness, health, and resilience that enables individuals and groups to respond to everyday and even extraordinary life events with equanimity and compassion. Relational wellness is essentially the cultivation and enhancement of covitality, well-being, and learning power.

The 4-R AI process shown in Figure 5.1 is designed to provide a framework that illustrates how inquiry grounded in connectedness and respectful relationships can foster relational wellness and learning power in ways that promote covitality, positive personal, organizational, and community change. The appreciative inquiry 4-R process and participatory inquiry process (Table 6.1 in Part II) shows how the 4-R AI process can be aligned with the PIP step-by-step approach to promoting positive school change via inquiry based on respectful relationships, participatory leadership, and action. The 4-R AI process involves:

1. *Relational Connection*—building respectful relationships and relational wellness by listening to the positive core in the many narratives within the organization. Relational connection begins by nurturing, practicing, modeling, and even teaching basic communication skills to everyone within learning organizations; the basic attending skills described by Ivey, Packard, & Ivey (2006) are easily adapted and adjusted if student advocates want to encourage more listening and empathy within their school. The key is to help create a community where everyone listens, listens, listens, and listens some more in order to enter each other's world and understanding. In other words, help as many people as possible live with a deep understanding that the way I see the world is not the only way to see that world. Each individual exists in an ecological context that offers multiple perspectives about what is. Basic attending skills are fundamental to promoting relational wellness because they begin with helping and teaching individuals how to listen to each other and to enter the world of the other with empathy and understanding. Learning power—individual and group capacities directed toward new knowledge, understandings, competencies, as well as the resilience to spring back from failure, with the help of tutors, mentors, teachers, and counselors. Covitality—individual and group capacities directed toward fostering multiple positive psychological traits in all students.

   Practicing mindful wonderment is important in establishing and maintaining relational connection (Lewis et al., 2010). Mindful wonderment is acting in a way to maintain open wonder and curiosity about possibilities for seeing, hearing, and even responding to others from a fresh perspective. Mindful wonderment promotes relational connection by encouraging practitioners to use appreciative inquiry, concentration, and mindfulness in everyday practice (Cooperrider & Whitney, 1999; Greason & Cashwell, 2009; Kabat-Zinn, 1994; Langer, 1989). Mindful wonderment is an expansive term used to position practitioners into not taking any preferred or monolithic position in their inquiry and listening; that is, mindful wonder fosters openness and flexibility. Mindful wonderment draws upon four schools of thought: (a) Langer's (1989) definition of mindfulness; (b) narrative counseling's use of curiosity (Monk et al., 1997); (c) philosopher Arne Naess' (2002) concept that ways of seeing and being in the world are influenced by profound wondering and the recognition that anything is possible; and (d) appreciative inquiry understanding that there is a positive core that can be tapped in any organization. Appreciative inquiry helps illuminate what brings life into work, relationships, and actions (Cooperrider & Whitney, 1999) and orients practitioners to avoid the usual pitfall of 'blame and drain' gossip that often dominates organizations when relational wellness and difficult dialogues are needed to promote change. Mindful wonder enables practitioners to remain focused on exploring strengths, the positive core that gives life to the organization, and promoting relational wellness.

2. *Relational Dialogue*—involves engaged inquiry and envisioning what might be by generating possibility dialogues with different stakeholders, and generating possibility narratives about what could be done. Possibility dialogues can begin with specific individuals, such as supervisors, or by invitation to small group meetings, or even to large groups. The point is to initiate conversations and dialogues about what might be and to imagine and dream about a better future, improved performance, shared vision, etc. Relational possibilities are an invitation to allies and all community members to dream and image ways to promote relational wellness within the organization. There is an attempt to look at and talk about possible pathways for promoting relational wellness. The relational possibilities phase attempts to build interactional participation among stakeholders and to invite collaboration, consultation, and collective action toward group or organizational goals. This phase attempts to affirm that we are not alone and that we can build meaning together (Keltner, 2009). Together we will stand and work to reach for or to help an individual reach for a goal that is defined as the first step or action toward doing one thing differently. We will participate in a cycle of inquiry to improve current conditions.

3. *Relational Action*—must be relational in nature as it is directed toward joining with others to promote student and school community well-being and learning power. This phase involves actions being taken to compose new stories in the organization. Relational action transforms the possibility of what might be into this is what we are going to do to make our dream into clear, concrete, specific, and measurable goal(s). Relational action requires taking more responsibility and making a commitment to taking the first well-defined step in the change process. It also means defining the specific actions in a way that progress toward the goal can be assessed; what step are we on in the nine-step PIP? Goals, timelines, and responsibilities are defined. Dialogues shift to inviting collaborations, allies, and friends to commit to specific responsibilities in acting or supporting the goal. Who is going to do what, when?

4. *Relational Assessment and Reflection*—focuses on the rational telling and sharing of the new narrative, as well as getting feedback in order to keep nurturing the evolution and development of the living story. Relational assessment and reflection is about keeping the change effort rolling and seeing what the first step or doing one thing differently actions have resulted in. Where are we in relation to the goal? What is different? What has improved? What went well? Such questions mean seeking feedback and assessing clear, specific, and concrete goals. It is

recommended that the change process be documented and shared with stakeholders and other interested parties via a paper, presentation, posting, or other venue. You want to hear from students and their families. How has this action improved their experience in the school community? What we dreamed and imagined, and what happened are important aspects of any developmental activity. The point is to celebrate the learning power of the group and organization; and to assert that the collective supports individuals or engages in dreaming about ways to make things better for all students.

The documentation should also include reflection and recommendations for next steps. Change is not about waving a magic wand but patient and persistent effort to bring about desired results. The AI 4-R process and PIP require commitment. Patience may emanate from the relational aspect of the process, as participatory inquiry demands persistence. The 4-R describes "how" the community engages in the work while PIP outlines the steps to address "what" challenge is identified. The AI 4-R process reminds participants to focus on the school community's strengths and assets as well as perceived challenges. The desired results in this process are focused on fostering relational wellness in the organization, which is the next section.

Relational Wellness

Relational wellness is an overarching construct. Relational wellness results from what Prilleltensky and Prilleltensky (2006) refer to as synergy that connects three sites of well-being: personal, organizational, and community. In this text relational wellness is an umbrella term that includes covitality, learning power, and school connectedness. At the same time, relational wellness is ecological in that it is bound to the personal, organizational (school), and community, just as Prilleltensky and Prilleltensky's (2006) three primary sites of well-being asserts that well-being is not located in a singular site; well-being emerges from personal, organizational, and community sites. As a state of cognitive, emotional, and spiritual happiness, health, and resilience, well-being enables personal, organizational, and community responses to everyday and even extraordinary life events to be guided by a sense of equanimity and compassion.

Relational wellness is about the ecological vibrancy and life of ecosystems where people exist as learning beings—personally, in schools, and in communities at the same time. To concentrate on personal wellness and ignore school and community wellness is to lose the point. In this text, wellness, well-being, and covitality are bound together in an ecological understanding described as relational wellness. The point is that individual students exist in families, schools, neighborhoods, and communities that are embedded ecologically in relationship to each other. The health of one impacts the other; the three primary sites for where relational wellness will be framed in this text are personal, school, and community.

In Table 5.1, relational wellness is tied to resilience theory (Benard, 2004), learning power (Claxton, 2002), covitality (Furlong et al., 2013), and the Construct-Based Approach (Squier et al., 2014). The core constructs of these approaches converge in four domains aligned with relational wellness; the effort is a heuristic attempt to draw out what is common in each rather than assert that the theories are perfectly aligned.

Four Relational Wellness Discourse Domains

The four relational wellness discourse domains found in Table 5.1 could be cultivated and promoted in the school discourse. The domains can be used to guide students (personal), defined as core dispositions regarding what is taught in schools (school), and as essential qualities in the community (community). The discourse domains are designed to align with current theories but primarily to promote dialogue and discourse:

- *Performative Focus Discourse*: begins with talking about performance as an active art form. "Performative" as a term is related to dramatic or artistic performance. Personal and social competence are performative arts; interpersonal communication is performative; active efforts must be made to teach, play, or model listening, speaking, responding respectfully and directly. There is an attempt to teach, play, model, and build empathy for others, as well as care for self, family, school, and community. Students explore core concepts such as altruism, compassion, forgiveness, responsibility, loyalty, initiative, play, etc. This domain is connected to the Learning Power's Resilience construct that calls on educators to teach youth to cultivate personal absorption, managing distractions, noticing and perseverance (Claxton et al., 2011). This domain is also connected to the covitality Emotional Competence construct that is measured by one's skills at emotional regulation, self-control, and empathy (Furlong et al., 2013). This domain most aligned with the Motivation construct defined in the Construct-Based Approach (CBA) (Squier et al., 2014). This domain is roughly aligned with Benard's (2004) Matrix of Personal Strengths domain: Social Competence.
- *Vital Engagement Discourse*: begins with talking about engaged decision making, choice, and sense of control in a given situation; active effort must be made to teach students basic decision making skills, an appreciation for the complexity of the decision making process (Kahneman, 2011), and the importance of knowing an actor-centered, adaptive decision making process (Goldberg, 2001). It is crucial to engage and teach students resourcefulness, flexibility, planning, critical thinking, and how to trust and question their insight or intuition

(Benard, 2004; Claxton, 1997). It is equally important to simply play with no goal other than enjoyment and connection with others in the moment. This domain is connected to the Learning Power's Resourcefulness construct that calls on educators to teach youth to cultivate questioning, capitalizing, making links, reasoning, and imagining skills (Claxton et al., 2011). Furlong et al. (2013) define this domain as Engaged Living that is measured by one's optimism, zest, and gratitude. This domain is most aligned with the Self-Direction construct defined in the Construct-Based Approach (CBA) (Squier et al., 2014). This domain is roughly aligned with Benard's (2004) Matrix of Personal Strengths domain: Problem Solving.

- *Self-Reflectiveness Discourse*: begins with talking about reflective learning power and recognizing one's own sense of competence or at least an "island of competence" (Brooks & Goldstein, 2001). It builds upon resilience, resourcefulness, reflectiveness, and reciprocity (Claxton, 2002). Talking about learning power and the autonomy it provides may foster students' positive identity, internal locus of control, sense of self-efficacy, mastery, competence, and self-awareness, as well as greater capacity for adaptive distancing, mindfulness, and humor (Benard, 2004; Claxton, 1997, 2002). This domain is connected to the Learning Power's Resilience construct that calls on educators to teach youth to cultivate reflectiveness by planning, meta-learning, distilling, and revising (Claxton et al., 2011). This domain lines up with what Furlong et al. (2013) call Belief in Self as determined by one's self-awareness, self-efficacy, and grit. This domain most aligned with the Self-Knowledge construct defined in the CBA (Squier et al., 2014). This domain is roughly aligned with Benard's (2004) Matrix of Personal Strengths domain: Autonomy.

- *Relational Connectedness Discourse*: begins with connection to family, community, the physical environment, and purpose. It comes from the feeling that what is being done is meaningful, be it working toward a specific goal, learning something new, doing something playful, or even making sense of one's own life. Personally, sense of purpose can be tied to special interests, such as learning to play a musical instrument, developing one's creativity or imagination. Learning to play a musical instrument takes discipline, whereas imagining creatures in the clouds does not; but each has a purpose in the moment. Sense of purpose can range from having a role on a team to helping a grandparent rebuild an old car. In school, sense of purpose has to do with having the educational aspirations to meet the high expectations defined in every class. Sense of purpose calls forth hope and optimism, and is frequently tied to faith, spirituality, and finding a sense of meaning in life. This domain is connected to the Learning Power's Reciprocity construct that calls on educators to teach youth to cultivate imitation, interdependence, empathy, listening, and collaboration (Claxton et al.,

Table 5.1 Aligning Theories and Discourse Practices that Promote Learning Power and Wellness

	Performative Focus	Vital Engagement*	Self-Reflectiveness	Relational Connectedness
Lewis & Winkelman (2014) Relational Wellness Matrix Aligning Theories and Discourse Practices	**Discourse** • Personal/emotional competence • Social competence • Embodied competence • Play	**Discourse** • Decision making • Gratitude/thanks • Gumption • Grit • Bricolage (making do) • Play	**Discourse** • Reflective Learning Power • Making connections • Equanimity • Goals/results	**Discourse** • Peers, family • Adults, community • Physical environment • Purpose • Compassion • Play
Claxton et al. (2011) Building Learning Power (p. 17)	**Resilience** • Absorption • Managing distractions • Noticing • Perseverance	**Resourcefulness** • Questioning • Capitalizing • Making links • Reasoning • Imagining	**Reflectiveness** • Planning • Meta-learning • Distilling • Revising	**Reciprocity** • Imitation • Interdependence • Empathy and listening • Collaboration
Furlong et al.(2013) Covitality	**Emotional Competence** • Emotional regulation • Self-control • Empathy	**Engaged Living** • Optimism • ZEST • Gratitude	**Belief in Self** • Self-awareness • Self-efficacy • Grit	**Belief in Others** • Family coherence • Peer support • School support
Squier et al. (2014) Construct-Based Approach (p. 52)	**Motivation** • Describe how their own motivation structure and patterns affect their current and future lives • Articulate a positive vision of their future that motivates present behavior • Consistently apply effective self-motivational techniques	**Self-Direction** • Assess the factors responsible for their academic success and challenges and adjust their behavior accordingly • Demonstrate the self-direction, initiative and skills necessary for achievement and success • Maintain focus despite stress, anxiety and setbacks	**Self-Knowledge** • Describe how their unique characteristics impact their current and future lives • Demonstrate how their skills and talents contribute to their success • Discuss how their values and interests inform their decisions and actions	**Relationships** • Engage in collaborative and mutually beneficial relationships to promote individual and group success • Assess when they need help from others and seek assistance • Demonstrate fairness, respect, and equity in relationships with others
Benard (2004) Personal Strengths Matrix (p. 119)	Social Competence	Problem Solving	Autonomy	Sense of Purpose

Source: Lewis & Winkelman (2014)

2011). Furlong et al. (2013) define the relational wellness domain as Belief in Others as enhanced by family coherence, peer support, and school support. This domain is most aligned with the Relationships construct defined in the Construct-Based Approach (CBA) (Squier et al., 2014). This domain is roughly aligned with Benard's (2004) Matrix of Personal Strengths domain: Purpose/Future.

Csikszentmihalyi and Nakamura use "vital engagement" to show that every path is a unique opportunity to experience moments of flow (enjoyed absorption) doing what is focused upon. "Vital engagement" is another way of saying that the action enabled the individual to enact "love made visible" (see Haidt, 2006, p. 224). For Furlong et al., see: www.michael furlong.info/web_hppis2e_covitality_chap.pdf

There are alternative ways to frame relational wellness, such as the ASCA *Mindsets and behaviors for student success* (ASCA, 2014) mentioned earlier, or the Collaborative for Academic, Social and Emotional Learning's (CASEL) simple five core social emotional competencies (www.casel.org/basics/skills.php):

1. self-awareness—being able to accurately assess one's feelings, interests, values, and strengths; maintaining a well-grounded sense of self-confidence;
2. self-management—being able to regulate one's emotions to handle stress, control impulses, and persevere in overcoming obstacles; setting and monitoring progress toward personal and academic goals; expressing emotions appropriately;
3. social awareness—being able to take the perspective or point of view of others and empathize with them; recognizing and appreciating individual and group similarities and differences; recognizing and using family, school, and community resources;
4. relationship skills—being able to establish and maintain healthy and rewarding relationships based on cooperation; resisting inappropriate social pressure; preventing, managing, and resolving interpersonal conflict; seeking help when needed;
5. responsible decision making—being able to make decisions based on consideration of ethical standards, safety concerns, appropriate social norms, respect for others, and likely consequences of various actions; applying decision making skills to academic and social situations; contributing to the well-being of one's school and community.

There are also efforts such as the ASCD's Whole Child Initiative that is promoting students' long-term development and success by changing education policy and practice. Their approach to meeting the comprehensive needs of all students involves the shared responsibility of students, families, schools, and communities in five Whole Child Tenets:

1. Each student enters school healthy and learns about and practices a healthy lifestyle.
2. Each student is learning in an environment that is physically and emotionally safe for students and adults.
3. Each student is actively engaged in learning and is connected to the school and the broader community.
4. Each student has access to personalized learning and is supported by qualified, caring adults.
5. Each student is challenged academically and prepared for success in college or further education and for employment and participation in a global environment (www.ascd.org/whole-child.aspx).

The point in sharing these diverse constructs is to help expose the overlap, and hopefully, the alignment, of the theories. As human constructs, each offers perspectives that can be aligned with skill development in order to frame strengths-based interventions concerned with developmental resilience and living life with a sense of well-being and learning power. The constructs do not have to be in competition, but some wellness constructs may be better suited for some contexts than others. Relationships and dialogues built in phase 1 of either PIP or AI will help determine the constructs you choose to guide your conversations.

The 4-R AI process provides a framework for initiating inquiry grounded in connectedness and respectful relationships that foster relational wellness and learning power in ways that promote the constructs described in Table 5.1. Below is a Reflective Moment that concentrates on using AI to explore the positive core of: performative focus, vital engagement, self-reflectiveness, and relational connections.

Reflective Moment 5.2

This is a reflective moment that has you reflect on four categories of relational wellness. It could be adapted to address any of the constructs found in Table 5.1: Aligning Theories and Discourse Practices that Promote Learning Power and Wellness.

Relational Wellness Appreciative Inquiry Interview Protocol

1. Think of a time in your entire experience in school communities when you felt most excited, most engaged, and most alive. What were the *performative focus* factors that made it a great experience? What was it about you that gave you a sense of personal/emotional competence, social competence, or even a sense of embodied competence?

2. What connects you to your work and helps you feel a sense of *vital engagement* in what you are doing in your school community? Do you feel engaged in decision making? Are there experiences and relationships you have gratitude for or feel thanks for? Has the program prompted you into having the gumption to do something you thought you could not do? Has the program helped you learn how to make do with what you have? Does the program liberate you to play more?

3. In what ways has your *self-reflectiveness* been enhanced? Have you recognized a reflective learning power, where you notice that you "got it" with a challenging concept or skill? Have you made connections with your school community experiences and your current sense of purpose? Have you been able to take a perspective that enables you to look at a problem with equanimity? Have you been able to define goals and look at your personal results in your movement toward those goals?

4. In what ways have your *relational connections* been enhanced? Do you feel more connection with peers and family? With older adults and within the community? A special connection to the physical environment? A deeper sense of purpose? More willingness to play? More compassion for others?

Based on: Ludema, Cooperrider, & Barrett (2000).

AI Focus Groups, Fishbowl Groups and Summits

Appreciative inquiry takes what has been described above and invites professionals to cultivate their own positive core in order to enhance their own performative focus, vital engagement, self-reflectiveness, and relational connections. Inquiry and mindful wonderment are used to enrich what the Dalai Lama calls "compassionate moral responsibility" in order to be a "force for good" (Goleman, 2015). The purpose of AI in schools is to cultivate the positive core. To achieve this purpose, professionals begin by enhancing their own positive core and relational wellness, in order to work with individuals, groups, and in school systems. They also recognize that appreciative inquiry builds from collaborating with others and fostering a learning community. Appreciative inquiry summits involve entire departments and expand to school-wide meetings that concentrate on cultivating the positive core. Planning and preparation are vital to any successful AI summit. School administrators, department chairs, and other key leaders must be engaged in the process leading up to an AI summit. That is why sometimes it is best to begin with a focus group or fishbowl group with students. The students are an important resource for exploring the positive core at any school.

Focus groups or fishbowl groups are designed to deepen conversations about the positive core in the school and to explore possibilities for enhancing relational wellness, learning power, or any of the constructs described previously. The point is that those leading AI groups must be grounded in the positive core and relational wellness constructs, and allies and school leaders must be informed and included, if possible. Group leaders need structure and the ability to improvise. Focus group and fishbowl group leaders are guided by AI interview protocols, such as that found in Reflective Moment 5.2. More practical guidelines for focus, fishbowl, and even video recording groups will be offered in Part II.

Advocacy and Participatory Leadership

Appreciative inquiry and the 4-R AI process require that advocates act as participatory leaders who know how to build relationships, actively listen, align dreams, create learning communities where there are opportunities to participate and contribute, provide members with room to exercise their own discretion in how they will be involved, and act positively about future possibilities for the school. Crucial to framing change is the student advocate's understanding of the need to promote relational wellness throughout the school and to model continuous development in the wellness domains: performative focus, vital engagement, self-reflectiveness, and relational connectedness. The advocate can cultivate relational wellness by presenting workshops and embodying practices that are guided by the 4-R AI process: 1) relational connection, 2) relational dialogue, 3) relational action, and 4) relational assessment and reflection.

Chapter Summary

This chapter offers three lifescaping practices that can inform strengths-based change: appreciative inquiry, the appreciative inquiry 4-R process, and the four relational wellness domains. Appreciative inquiry (AI) focuses upon and builds upon the existing positive core that exists in any organization, especially schools. AI offers the conceptual frame for moving conversations and inquiry toward expanding upon the positive core. The chapter shares that AI has eight strengths-based principles: 1) the constructionist principle, 2) the principle of simultaneity, 3) the poetic principle, 4) the anticipatory principle, 5) the positive principle, 6) the wholeness principle, 7) the ethical enactment principle, and 8) the free choice principle. The principles help participatory leaders deepen the understanding of the positive core throughout the school in ways that introduce new language and ways of modeling the wellness domains and integrating the appreciative inquiry 4-R process into everyday practice. The 4-R AI process is a continuous cycle that moves and repeats this living course of action: 1) relational connection, 2) relational dialogue, 3) relational action, and 4) relational assessment and reflection. Participatory leaders are encouraged to develop and model the qualities described as wellness domains: performative focus, vital engagement, self-reflectiveness, and relational connectedness.

In Part II, Chapters 6–9, the four phases of PIP and AI are presented individually in chapters and sequentially in order to help advocates and site administrators to take steps to integrate strengths-based ecological practices into their future forming efforts at their schools.

Part II

Lifescaping as Future Forming

From an Appreciative Inquiry
Approach to Enacting the
Participatory Inquiry Process

Introduction

Part II details the four AI and PIP phases described in Chapter 4 and
Chapter 5. The appreciative inquiry 4-R process and participatory inquiry
process (Table 6.1) are designed to help advocates make connections
between the PIP described in Chapter 4 and the AI 4-R process described
in Chapter 5.

In Part II, we concentrate on offering sequential actions, and moving
through the phases and steps introduced and described in the previous
Chapters 4 and 5. It is important to note with both PIP and the 4-R AI
process, advocates should be ready to step back to an earlier phase or step
if necessary. What is described in linear and sequential step-by-step terms
is actually a recursive process that loops back when necessary. Go slow,
build relationships and understandings before pushing forward. At the same
time, sometimes advocates must put themselves on the line, develop a small
measurable project on their own to illustrate PIP. Other times advocates
must take the risk to stand up and speak truth to oppressive power, and
be willing to be fired for the right and just cause. Even in the dramatic act,
it is important to recognize sometimes small wins over time are much more
powerful than self-absorbed acts where the individual goes out in flames
of glory. This work involves having the courage to speak truth to power
but we think building inclusive and diverse groups with a vision and the
willingness to actively lifescape their local community is more powerful
than messianic leaders pushing an agenda that always seems to bend the
light in their direction. Participatory leadership includes other voices *and*
takes action that is reflected upon and adjusted in a never-ending growth
process within communities of practice.

PIP and AI are continuous forms of conditioning for maintaining a
growth mindset in your school community. The phases and steps guide

advocates with specific projects and intervention efforts within their schools and districts. Where are we now? What can we do? How do we move forward? PIP looks at the "*What* can we do to move forward in our future forming efforts?" AI explores the "*How* can we work from our positive core in our future forming efforts?" Each complements the other. The project guided by PIP may require an appreciative inquiry workshop to explore the positive core of the organization, whereas the project guided by AI might come to the point where individuals join together to examine a specific issue such as student truancy more deeply. Again, both PIP and AI are guided by a growth mindset, and advocates using either PIP or AI will make choices about what fits best in their local context.

Each of the next four chapters in Part II concentrates on one of the AI or PIP phases. Phase 1 of both PIP and AI are described in Chapter 6, Phase 2 in Chapter 7, Phase 3 in Chapter 8, and Phase 4 in Chapter 9. Table 6.1 lists the Appendices and Actions aligned with each chapter. The intention is to help guide readers so that they will be able to make the most use of the text and adjust their reading and use of the text to best fit their own needs as advocates in local settings. The four action research PIP phases and nine steps are described in the first column. The four AI phases are described in the second column. The third column lists the focus of the chapter and the actions that can be taken to deepen understanding or move the PIP or AI process to the next phase. The phases should not be viewed as linear and rigidly sequential, but should always be understood as looping back to build relationships and deepen dialogue and inquiry in order to define action. Once action has been taken, it is important to assess and reflect upon what occurred. Limitations and recommendations are explored in order to help the future forming actions remain alive.

Table 6.1 Participatory Inquiry Process (PIP) and Appreciative Inquiry (AI) 4-R Process

Participatory Inquiry Process (PIP) What? Overview Chapter 4	Appreciative Inquiry Process (4-R) How? Overview Chapter 5	Preparation Activities, Actions, and Reflections
Phase 1: Initiating Conversations and Identifying Challenges **Step 1.** Advocates begin the inquiry process by examining the school environment, accessible school data, and other school-wide sources of information that will begin to provide the school's narrative. **Step 2.** Advocates facilitate conversations, dialogues, and collaborations among community members to identify challenges.	**Phase 1: Relational Connection** is about building respectful relationships and relational wellness by listening to the positive core in the narratives within the organization. What is and is not working for students? From whose perspective?	**Action Focus: Chapter 6** Action Tools: • Complete Figure 6.1 and 6.2 • Activity 6.1 • Data Sheets (Appendix D) • PIP/AI Action Worksheet (Appendix I) • Review Appendix J
Phase 2: Engaged Inquiry **Step 3.** Using a variety of resources, dialogues and engaged inquiry are initiated to explore possibilities for responses to the challenge(s)being addressed. **Step 4.** Using available school-based data, baseline, comparative, and data trends are investigated and reflected upon by the learning community.	**Phase 2: Relational Dialogue** involves engaged inquiry and dreaming about what might be by generating possibility dialogues with different community members, and generating possibility narratives about what could be done.	**Action Focus: Chapter 7** • Driving and Restraining (Appendix G) • Parent Permission Form (Appendix F) • Needs Assessment (Appendix E)
Phase 3: Collaborative Action **Step 5.** Conversations about problems, challenges, and actions are directed toward defining meaningful, measurable, and realistic goals and strategies that address the challenge(s). **Step 6.** Actions are taken to put the agreed upon strategy(s) into practice.	**Phase 3: Relational Action** must be relational in nature as it is directed toward promoting student and school community well-being and learning power. This phase involves actions being taken to compose new narratives in the organization.	**Action Focus: Chapter 8** • Activities 8.1, 8.2, 7.3 • Focus and Fishbowl Groups (Appendix H) • Implement agreed upon lesson, intervention, etc.
Phase 4: Community Assessment and Reflection **Step 7.** Advocates assist in determining and providing venues for community assessment and reflection. **Step 8.** The strategy(s) is adapted accordingly via continuing learning community reflection. **Step 9.** Action is taken to put the revised strategy(s) into practice, and necessary steps are repeated.	**Phase 4: Relational Assessment and Reflection** focuses on the rational telling and sharing of the new narrative, as well as getting feedback in order to keep nurturing the evolution and development of the living story.	**Action/Reflection Focus: Chapter 9** • Reflect, share, and document • Outline for writing report (Appendix J) • Submit for publication • Revise the strategy to further improve outcome

6 Developing Relational Connections to Initiate Conversations and Identify Challenges

We come into life through relationship.

(Kenneth J. Gergen, 2009, p. 34)

There are two things that interest me: the relation of people to each other, and the relation of people to land.

(Nina Leopold, unpublished manuscript)

In Chapter 6, we explore in greater depth how to take action to enact AI Phase 1: Relational Connections and PIP Phase 1: Initiating Conversations and Identifying Challenges. Advocates and participatory leaders develop philosophical positions and professional orientations in order to effectively practice the art, science, and craft of teaching and learning with others. As educators, we begin by listening deeply, like anthropologists who are entering an unexplored culture and world. This book is arguing that relationships between and among people in human ecosystems, as well as the human relationship with life-giving ecosystems, is central to promoting learning and wellness. Educator advocates well-grounded in their professional practice act to balance protective factors: care and support, high expectations, and meaningful participation and contribution. Such practitioners reflect and act upon aspirational ethics and ethical guidelines to steer their day-to-day practice. They are part of educational communities of practice. They have a philosophical core yet remain open to theory, research, and practices that inform and transform their evolving practice. Each professional story has substance, and this chapter shows engaged educator advocates ways we can be open to innovative ideas for guiding our practice. Effective educator advocates try to see the world afresh and remove the scales of habit from their eyes. They listen deeply to the story being shared and work mindfully to not come to snap conclusions, judgments, or quick offers of advice. They understand that systemic inequities must be thoroughly examined from a position of mindful wonderment: Why is this so? There are no "quick fixes" to remedy the deep divides between the haves and the have nots; there is only a relentless effort to improve learning conditions for ALL students.

This chapter addresses how to look with an artist's eye in order to see and how to listen with a therapist's ear in order to hear, while recognizing that everything people experience is mediated through language, beliefs, social forces, etc. (Sturken & Cartwright, 2001; Taylor, 2012). Due to the reality of mediated experience, this chapter will provide tools for looking and listening to help you see and hear things from a certain, and hopefully, respectful and inclusive perspective at your school.

But first, it is important to look at your school setting (based on Ellis & Hughes, 2002).

Ecology of Place: Looking at School Setting

Seeing and Hearing Activity 6.1

Please take the time to write your responses to the questions in order to deepen how you look at your school setting and how the school setting might seem to students, teachers, administrators, parents, and other community members. Consider the implications of your responses for the students you serve.

In so far as it is possible, drive or walk around your school and ask yourself the following questions to help you see your school:

1. Look at houses in the neighborhood. What are they like? Are they well maintained? Bars on the windows? Gardens or plants? Aesthetically, what do you see? Describe what might be considered pleasing, beautiful, interesting, or eye-opening.
2. Look at the entire school campus. How are the boundaries defined? What are the borders and confines of the school? Are there fences? How high? Are they maintained? Are there recognized and defined entrances? Are their holes or spots in the fences where people enter and exit the school?
3. Look at the parking lot and parking area. Is there a specific parking lot for faculty and staff? Are there parking spaces reserved for visitors? How close is the visitor reserved parking to the main building entrance?
4. Look at the athletic fields or playgrounds. Are there grass playing fields? Are they maintained? How many baseball, soccer, football, or other playing fields are there? Are there play structures or field exercise equipment?

5. Look at the trees and shrubbery. Are there trees at the school? Is there a shrubbery? Are the different shrubs maintained? Are there spots where students might not be safe or where students can hide? Are there spots that cannot be carefully supervised?

6. Look at the school entrance or main building. Do you have any idea about its design? The architect? When was it built? How well is the building exterior maintained? Are there signs that help newcomers find their way into the school?

7. Look at the other school buildings. How many portable buildings are there? How long have the portables been in use? How well are the buildings maintained? Are there signs that help newcomers find their way around the school?

8. Look at the signage. How inviting are the signs into the school? How helpful are the signs indicating where and what places are in the school? Are the signs in English and the key languages spoken within the students' homes?

9. Look at the classrooms. Are the classrooms accessible to all students? What teaching equipment is in the classroom? Are there chalkboards with chalk, whiteboards with markers, large screen televisions, projectors for instruction, and computers for students? Are there defined smart rooms with internet access for the teacher and screens where the content can be projected for the students to see? Does the equipment work? Do the staff and faculty know how to use it? Describe the teaching materials. What types of tables, chairs, and desks are there? Are they in good repair? What about the light? Is there natural light as well as overhead light?

10. Restrooms. Are the restrooms clean? Adequate light? Doors on the toilet stalls? Are there soap dispensers, paper towels, and toilet paper? Is there graffiti?

11. Cafeteria. Do students dine in the cafeteria? Describe the eating areas: Are the tables and chairs/benches in good repair? Are the floors clean? Describe the food: Is there any food from the school farm or local sources? If students are around, note how the students group themselves in the cafeteria.

12. Hallways and classrooms. How busy and noisy is it in the hallways between and during class? Pushing? Is the noise a buzz of human exchange? Is the tone respectful or is swearing part of the passing exchange? When walking by classrooms in session, are they filled with life? Do the tone and exchanges sound engaged?

13. Blind spots. Are there areas on campus that are difficult to monitor? Who are the students who find these spots? What are some of the things that take place in these spots?
14. Library and computers. Does the library seem inviting, offering a "come on in" sort of feel as you look from the outside? Is the library accessible? Does it have abundant books and learning materials? Is there literature related to being or having parents who are gay, lesbian, bisexual? Are there materials related to the different students' ethnic heritage? Is there a computer room or easy student access to functional and up to date computers?
15. Family room. Is there a family room or community space that is reserved for families or community members who are part of the school community? Are there resources and materials made available to families and community members that would help them network with others in the community? Is there a family liaison?
16. Administration offices. Do the administration offices look inviting? What kinds of materials are posted on the walls, doors, etc.? Do the materials highlight anything special? Are posted materials in languages other than English? Is the district or school mission/vision clearly visible? Are school-wide awards, accreditation status, and other materials posted in plain view? Are there student photos? Are the student photos representative of the school's demographics/diversity? Do the secretaries or support personnel smile and/or greet individuals coming into the office? Do individual offices invite others to see the administrator as a person, i.e., family or vacation photos on table or wall. Are his/her degrees and credentials posted on the wall? Is there a separate room for meeting with families or as a small group?
17. Counseling, school psychology, school social work offices. Do the counseling, school psychology, and school social worker offices look inviting? What kinds of materials are posted on the walls, doors, etc.? Are there safe space posters? Are the SAT or ACT dates and school code posted in areas that are easy to see? Are posted materials in languages other than English? Is the school counseling program vision clearly visible? Are any goals and data posted? Are there student photos? Are the student photos representative of the school's demographics/diversity? Do the secretaries or support personnel smile and/or greet individuals coming into the office? Do individual offices invite others to see the counselor, school psychologist, or school social worker as a person, i.e., family or vacation photos on table or wall. Are his/her degrees and credentials posted on the wall?

Is there a separate room for meeting with families or as a small group? Does the counselor have a computer? What sort of data system do they use?

18. School health center. Is there a school-based health center? Do students have access to health care and dentistry on or near campus? Do students have access to a school nurse? Can students be easily referred to health care?

Personalizing the Organizational Structure of the District and School

Walking around the school and throughout the school community orients you to the physical environment where students come every day to learn. Human organizations also have explicit and implicit organizational structures that define certain individuals to act as leaders. Schools are no different. Figures 6.1 and 6.2 offer a generic organizational overview of school districts and schools. Figure 6.1 provides an overview of a school district. It is vital to see that public school districts generally have elected school boards who are responsible for overseeing the budget and how the district schools define and meet the local vision, mission, goals, and state educational mandates. School boards are also responsible to the community, even the most marginalized groups in the community. School boards hire school superintendents to act as the key educational leaders responsible for implementing the school board's policies. Assistant superintendents and other personnel report to the superintendent, as do school principals and other district personnel. Always bear in mind that the vision, mission, goals, policies, and state educational mandates should always focus on how best to help students learn to learn, learn to live, learn to work, and learn to contribute as productive citizens in a pluralistic democracy. That is the common language you will always have with school boards and district administrators. That is also why knowing the professional research in your field and having data about your school will help you engage and inform district leaders about how stakeholders can team and collaborate to help all students live up to meeting the vision, mission, goals, policies, and state educational mandates. This also means that educational professionals must speak out when the vision, mission, goals, and policies might not be in, or implemented in, ways that are in the best interests of all students.

The school board is the ultimate governing body of the school district. District superintendents and their assistants serve at the discretion of the school board, which is elected by the local population. School site principals

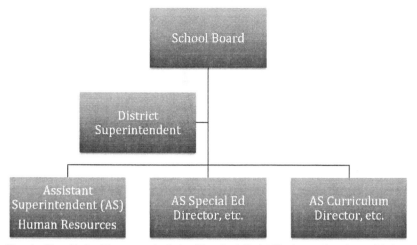

The school board is the ultimate governing body of the school district. District superintendents and their assistants serve at the discretion of the school board, which is elected by the local population. School site principals report to the district superintendent or to those district-level administrators appointed by the superintendent to supervise the site principals.

Figure 6.1 Generic District Organizational Structure

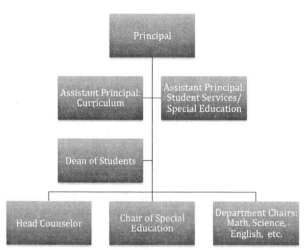

Each school has a principal and assistant principals who report to the district administration. The school board defines the district's vision, mission, and goals.

Figure 6.2 Generic School Organizational Structure

report to the district superintendent or to those district-level administrators appointed by the superintendent to supervise the site principals. Each school has a principal and assistant principals who report to the district administration. The school board defines the district's vision, mission, and goals.

Figure 6.2 shows the generic organizational chart for individual schools. Principals report to the superintendent, but the principals are the educational leaders who are appointed by school boards to implement and meet the board's vision, mission, goals, policies, and state educational mandates. Principals often designate a leadership team charged to help fulfill the board's vision, mission, goals, policies, and state educational mandates. As with district level administrators, the vision, mission, goals, policies, and state educational mandates should always focus on how best to help students learn to learn, learn to live, learn to work, and learn to contribute as productive citizens in a pluralistic democracy.

Seeing and Hearing Activity 6.2

Using Figures 6.1 and 6.2, align the position titles that are listed with the district and school where you are. Generally, school districts have organizational charts with this information. If the district or school organizational charts do not have names, place the names of the individuals next to their job titles. Attend or watch a broadcast of a school board meeting. Make sure you get the names of the school board members. Although this may difficult to do, and not even possible, be curious without being intrusive in learning about your school board representatives:

- Do they have children in school?
- Did they attend the local schools?
- What do they do professionally?
- What is their key interest in schools?

What seems to be their positions regarding students, the community, and the role of school? What do you observe in board meetings? Do individual members respond with statements and actions that demonstrate a belief that all children can learn and develop competencies?

The intention of your information gathering is to learn about school board members as people; it is not an effort to find embarrassing facts but to get to know their interests and motivations to help youth. You can use the same approach with the superintendent and other district leaders. Again, you are trying to get a sense of their vision of helping youth and serving as educational leaders.

If other administrative leaders at your school have the time, engage them in conversations based on Seeing and Hearing Activity 6.2. Department chairs and other school leaders should also be approached with similar questions and observations. Depending on your time, you want to generate conversations with a variety of leaders found on the school organizational chart (Figure 6.2). Remember, the intention is to learn more about them as people and educators, as well as their positive intentions for helping all students live up to their potential.

School Data and School Story

This section calls for you to get school data and information so that you can begin to create a school story based on the available data. You may find data in accreditation reports, district websites, school websites, state websites, and other sources. You may want to use the data templates in Appendix D and the prompts below to get yourself thinking about the richness of data within any school and district. The task of finding data is not always easy. In fact, it is impossible at times. Knowing this can help you advocate for having schools and districts keep and track certain kinds of data.

Seeing and Hearing Activity 6.3

Please complete the data templates in Appendix D. You might not be able to obtain all of the data, but get as much data as you are able to manage. This data will provide you with an objective and frequently powerful story that can be further examined through collaborative conversations with community members (teachers, students, parents, and other school-helping professionals).

The point is that the data shape the school's ecological narrative because individuals choose to look at and listen to data in certain areas while ignoring or simply not being aware of data they might not like. Counselors are well positioned to gather critical data concerning students' school experience. They may contribute informal data gathered from counseling conversations or they may conduct formal focus groups addressing relevant school issues and investigating possible actions.

Seeing and Hearing Activity 6.4

Please take the time to write your responses to the questions in order to define your own thinking about the questions and the perspective being raised in this text. Consider the implications of your responses for the students you serve as a professional. Look at the data from an academic perspective.

- What assessments are used to evaluate academic progress at the school?
- At each grade level, what are the percentile scores for the three most current assessments (see Appendix D for school data template)?

There is more to any school than mere academic scores and newsletters. Schools are complex learning communities where students are taught to learn about how to learn, live, and work among peers with the support of adult mentors and caretakers.

Reflective Moment 6.1

Please take the time to write your responses to the questions in order to define your own thinking about the questions and the perspective being raised in this text. Consider the implications of your responses for the students you serve as a professional. Look at the data from a personal/social perspective.

- Are there any social/emotional assessment results for students? Instruments such as the Social Emotional Health Survey, California Healthy Kids Survey, etc.?
  - Does the school assess social emotional development? If so, are there comparative scores over a three-year period? If not, are there any measures for or documentation of student development in these areas not typically assessed:
    - Decision making skills?

- Social competence?
- Sense of autonomy, i.e., positive identity, internal locus of control, initiative, self-efficacy, etc. (Benard, 2004)?
- Sense of purpose, i.e., goal direction, educational aspirations, creativity, special interests, etc. (Benard, 2004)?

- What do the assessment data say about the academic and social/emotional character of the school?
  - Is the school below average, average, or above average academically? According to what measures?
  - What is the evidence that the school has high expectations for all students?
  - Is the school below average, average, above average in terms of social/emotional education?
  - What is the evidence that the school offers care and support for all students?
  - Are there any data that show students have meaningful opportunities to contribute to their school? What are the sources of that data? What are the activities and opportunities?

Schools create stories about themselves. They have themes, i.e., "We are an academic school and our standardized test scores are in the top five percent," etc. What is the theme at your school? What does your program support?

Reflective Moment 6.2

Please take the time to write your responses to the questions in order to define your own thinking about the questions and the perspective being raised in this text. Consider the implications of your responses for the students you serve as a professional. Look at the data for themes and your own program development perspective. There might not be data but you are being challenged to explore and think about these topics.

- What perspective or point of view does the school have regarding whether the students:
  - understand that there are clear high expectations for all;
  - feel that adults at the school care and support them in reaching those high expectations;

- – are able to find opportunities for meaningful participation and contribution to their school or community?
- Are the adults and students oriented to a growth mindset toward learning, where they understand that they have "learning muscles" rather than fixed abilities?
- How often and in what format(s) are students asked about their school experience?
- How would you describe the theme of the data and information above? How would you frame that description so that you could share it with community members at your site?
- Describe some aspect of your school setting, either inside or outside of the building, that students might be able to do to improve how the school looks.
- Find or develop a list of the activities and programs that the school has to address academic and personal/social challenges for all students. List the name of the program, the population it is designed to serve, the grade levels served, and the specific activities it offers.
  - – Are there any programs or activities you might be able to build on, participate in, or even create to help students connect to school more effectively?
- School Counseling Program
  - – Is there a comprehensive school counseling program based on the *ASCA national model* (2012)?
  - – Are there a program mission statement and a vision statement that focus on all students' success?
  - – Are there program goals that define how the mission and vision are to be measured?
  - – Are there any school-wide student competencies related to the school counseling program?
  - – Has a school counseling program audit been conducted (see ASCA, 2012)?
  - – Has there been research conducted to assess any part of the school counseling program?
- School Psychology Program and Services
  - – How do school psychologists provide consultation and education to teachers and parents about learning disabilities and strategies for learning?
  - – Is there a positive behavior intervention system or school-wide plan to support clear expectations and a positive school climate?
  - – Are there any school-wide student competencies related to the school psychology program and services?
- Has a program audit been conducted?

Listening to Individual Stories at School

Reflective Moment 6.3

In Reflective Moment 6.3, you will find guidelines for exploring different stories about your school. For this activity, engage three to five individuals associated with your school in a dialogue about their school story. The conversation protocol in 6.3 follows the basic elements of any story. Please take the time to record the responses as accurately as possible. Also, reflect upon the implications of what is being shared. It is important to listen without judgment, and to listen to learn. Consider the implications of your responses for the students you serve as a professional.

This next activity calls for you to interview three to five different individuals associated with your school. You are trying to understand the basic elements to their narratives about the school where you work. Make sure that one of the people you talk with is an administrator, department or program chair, or other appointed leader at your site. You might even want to consult with him/her in choosing the other individuals with whom you will have conversations. The point is to try to engage in dialogue with diverse individuals, such as an administrator, a teacher, a parent, a counselor, a school psychologist, a student, a secretary, etc. to gain different perspectives.

Reflective Moment 6.4

- Plot (vision, mission, etc.)
  - Given your experience at school, what can you tell me about a highpoint or exceptional experience?
  - How does the school address developing the potential of all students? Have you discussed a growth mindset, the notion that learning muscles can be exercised to help students develop to their greatest potential?
  - What do they think the vision or mission of the school or school counseling program is?
  - What does public education mean to you? What do you believe is, or should be, the goal of public education?
  - More specifically, how could a comprehensive school counseling program help all students?

- Character (role)
    - What is your role or title at school?
    - How do you share your insights within the organization?
    - What do you do to make sure that you listen to those who have less social capital and may be marginalized to get their insights or solutions to everyday problems or challenges?
    - What is or has been the most positive and exciting thing you have been able to do since you came to the school?
    - When have you felt most successful in terms of your contributions to the school?
- Perspective/Point of View
    - What is the most life-enhancing aspect of the work being done at this school?
    - How does the school help students improve their decision making abilities?
    - What traditions or things that we are doing should be preserved as changes are made to the school or student services program?
    - What has been most nurturing for you as a member of the school community?
- Theme
    - If you could say there is a school theme, what theme is being played out at school? Athletic traditions? Academic excellence? Problem saturated environment?
    - How are the students at school labeled or grouped by adults? By their peers?
    - Are there educators whose basic orientation toward students falls into growth mindset versus fixed mindset positions? How do their professional themes play out at school?
    - How would people in the community describe our school theme?
    - How would the school board describe our school theme?
- Setting
    - Talk about our school as a place. Describe the outside and inside of the building.
    - What do you like best about our school setting?
    - Do you have a favorite spot to sit, watch students, or just relax?
- Challenges
    - What do you see as our three greatest challenges at school?
    - What programs do we have in place for addressing those challenges?
    - What do you see as our goal for this year?

- What is the first step to take toward that goal?
- Who do you need help from in reaching that goal?
- At the end of the school year, what would you like to be able to say about how we met at least one of the challenges you described?
- Describe a time when someone went out of their way to help you address a challenge or problem you were facing at school. What made it possible for them to help?

Mapping School and Community Assets

The data above and other resources can be used to develop asset maps of both the school and the community. Finding out what the school and community resources are is vital to constructing a collaborative change effort (Griffin & Farris, 2010). The data generated in the text can be used as a starting point for listing and mapping resources at school and the community that are assets supporting student learning power and wellness. School clubs and opportunities for students are just two examples. The key is that it is important to map both school and community assets. Where is the linkage? School and community asset maps will help clarify possible allies and resources. Such mapping may help define and can certainly be aligned with the defined challenge to be addressed.

Seeing and Hearing Activity 6.5

Develop an asset map of your school and community. List what is right with your school. What are its strengths? Try to find links. List allies and resources.

Explore a Possible Challenge to Be Addressed

You have learned about the ecological perspective, appreciative inquiry, the 4-R process, gathered data, and listened to stories about the strengths and challenges within your school. At this point, you want to create a list of possible challenges you can address, given your skills, position, social capital, and the assets you can engage/draw upon in your community. The next chapter will help you narrow your list, talk with colleagues, students, families, leaders, and community members to begin to shape an action pathway for you to collaboratively build and follow. The list can consist of challenges; it can also consist of assets that you want to build upon in order to improve the results of actions taking place to address specific challenges at school.

Seeing and Hearing Activity 6.6

Phase 1: Initiating Conversations and Identifying Challenges

PIP Step 1. The student advocate begins the inquiry process by examining the school environment, accessible school data, and other school-wide sources of information that will begin to tell the school's story. Student advocates enter the community like an anthropologist by listening to individuals and groups to hear some of the school's stories and story elements, including such characteristics as the school's strengths, assets, and perceived challenges as a learning community. The school-helping professional will begin to (collaboratively) define how to lifescape the school with others or to respond to a challenge that has been defined.

Reflective PIP Activity: Please describe some part of your school that you would like to lifescape with others; what would you like to do? Or list the challenges confronting students in your school that you want to consider addressing. Also, list student, program, and community assets that you might build upon to improve the results of actions taking place at your school. Consider who should be engaged in conversations about defining the lifescape you want to create or talking about the challenges you observe.

Initiating Conversations and Identifying Challenges: Questions to Consider

Reflective Moment 6.5

- What are your program or school's strengths?
- How do students describe the support offered at your school? What is working for them and what is not? Why? What suggestions do they have?
- How do families, other helping professionals, teachers, and community members describe the support offered to students at your

school? What is working and what is not? Why? What suggestions do they have?
- What have others done effectively? Elsewhere?
- Where did the program(s) come from?
- What are some possible directions that could be taken to promote student well-being and success?
- What is something that you would like to do to enhance the school's learning and well-being lifescape?
- What's a first step?

Initial Literature Review

As you move forward in your conversations about identifying your lifescape vision or the challenge to be addressed, it is very important to consider the professional literature regarding the topic you choose. When stating professional literature, we mean peer-reviewed journals, texts, and other critical resources. Wikipedia is nice to get a rough idea, but a university library database, journals, and materials are going to offer content that is less subject to whim and distortion than much of what can be found merely on the internet. Although we do offer a number of useful, and even remarkable, website addresses as resources, the point here is that exploring the literature and listening to what others are doing in a variety of settings will help define and shape your project. Knowing the literature will also help you see that you are always standing on the shoulders and ideas of others. Knowledge gets generated by communities over time; knowledge is not so much about what is in your head as an individual but what is accessible to you as a thinking person, shared, and used in the community where you practice. Most the professional literature will speak about successful projects and interventions; rarely are the noble failures described from a position of learning or celebrated as models to guide practice. Still, our position is that those engaging in lifescaping and future forming should always view their practice in terms of learning and development. Taking such a position can reduce the anxiety and need to get it perfect. We are guided by bricolage and makeshift acts as we learn and develop our professional craft. This is not haphazard; it is opening us to learning by doing. Knowing the literature helps one see the more successful pathways that have been followed or developed.

Planning Ahead for Publication

Before getting too far into your action research, think about publishing and think about the format you are going to use to share your work.

Remember, when making reports to your school and district, you want to use the name of your school. When publishing, you want to change the name of your school. When considering publication, it is very important to:

1. Change the name of your school, district, and individuals. For instance, "The names of the individuals, school, district, and community have been changed to respect the confidentiality of those participating in this study."
2. Change the name and generalize the location and size of the city, town or community.
   a. The National Center for Education Statistics Definitions (https://nces.ed.gov/surveys/ruraled/definitions.asp):
      i. City, Large: Territory inside an urbanized area and inside a principal city with population of 250,000 or more.
      ii. City, Midsize: Territory inside an urbanized area and inside a principal city with population less than 250,000 and greater than or equal to 100,000.
      iii. City, Small: Territory inside an urbanized area and inside a principal city with population less than 100,000.
      iv. Suburb, Large: Territory outside a principal city and inside an urbanized area with population of 250,000 or more.
      v. Suburb, Midsize: Territory outside a principal city and inside an urbanized area with population less than 250,000 and greater than or equal to 100,000.
      vi. Suburb, Small: Territory outside a principal city and inside an urbanized area with population less than 100,000.
      vii. Town, Fringe: Territory inside an urban cluster that is less than or equal to 10 miles from an urbanized area.
      viii. Town, Distant: Territory inside an urban cluster that is more than 10 miles and less than or equal to 35 miles from an urbanized area.
      ix. Town, Remote: Territory inside an urban cluster that is more than 35 miles from an urbanized area.
      x. Rural, Fringe: Census-defined rural territory that is less than or equal to 5 miles from an urbanized area, as well as rural territory that is less than or equal to 2.5 miles from an urban cluster.
      xi. Rural, Distant: Census-defined rural territory that is more than 5 miles but less than or equal to 25 miles from an urbanized area, as well as rural territory that is more than 2.5 miles but less than or equal to 10 miles from an urban cluster.
      xii. Rural, Remote: Census-defined rural territory that is more than 25 miles from an urbanized area and is also more than 10 miles from an urban cluster.

For instance, if talking about a city such as San Francisco, you might say, "This study takes place in a large city in Northern California with a population of approximately 300,000." If talking about the city of Albany, you might say, "This study takes place in a small suburb in the San Francisco Bay region with a population of approximately 80,000. In this study, I will refer to the community as Happy Acres in order to respect the confidentiality of those participating."

Publishing Venues

There are also a number of venues for publishing action research, such as the Social Publishers Foundation: www.socialpublishersfoundation.org/publish/. There is also the Action Research in School Counseling publishing page: www.schoolcounselor-advocate.com/#!projects/cfvg. Also, the Taos Institute has been instrumental in publishing open access materials as WorldShare publications. See Dole et al. (2014) who are the story curators for the Taos publication: *Exceeding expectations: An anthology of appreciative inquiry stories in education from around the world*. The text is open access and *Exceeding expectations* is a great resource for stories about how appreciative inquiry has had an impact on schools around the world. Efforts are currently under way to define a WorldShare open-access book that would publish lifescaping and future forming practices in schools in various regions of the United States. The Lifescaping Project can be contacted at lifescapingproject@gmail.com.

There is an Outline for writing 12–20 page action research (Appendix J) to help those who simply need a format to follow in writing about their action research PIP or AI projects. The outline provides one format that might be used to guide the writing process; it should be viewed as flexible and adaptable, not as a singular way of documenting the work.

Advocacy and Participatory Leadership

In order to initiate Phase 1 of the PIP or AI, participatory leaders are advised to reflect on the four skill-sets described in the wellness domain: performative focus, vital engagement, self-reflectiveness, and relational connectedness. All four skill-sets are necessary to be successful in Phase 1 of PIP and AI. Performative focus calls for personal and social competence via role play, practice, and other avenues. Advocates are required to look and listen deeply to what is happening in their school. Having the vital engagement or gumption—courage and confidence—necessary to see, hear, and ask questions to get data about their school is vital. Being self-reflective and able to make connections between the data and the students they see and hear is important, too. Learning about the essential value of relational connections throughout the school and community where they work is critical. Understanding and having compassion for those who do not have a voice is essential. Participatory leaders must be keenly aware of looking and listening in order to learn, rather than merely confirming "what is" or "what is told by others." Be alert to personalize people who make up the organization by getting to know about the person behind the job title. Reflect on the data, and wonder about such things as "Are the only data we use the academic data? Where are the data assessing personal/social well-being?" Participatory leaders seek out and listen to school narratives from diverse community members. Participatory leaders map the school's assets and explore the positive core in order to lifescape the school into a better place for all students.

Chapter Summary

This chapter challenges advocates and participatory leaders to begin with the artist's eye and ear, maintaining an appreciation for seeing and hearing about the positive core that exists. Being able to do these requires the wellness domain skill-sets of performative focus, vital engagement, and relational connections. Next, advocates are presented with data collection tools to help them to look and hear more deeply about the school, to get to know the people behind the roles, to reflect on the data about the school, and to understand the need to build on existing strengths. Being able to do these requires the wellness domain skill-set of self-reflectiveness, which draws upon both a sense of purpose and compassion for others. The chapter explores ways to fathom the school narratives and ways to initiate mapping the school's assets, exploring challenges to be addressed at the school, reviewing the necessary literature that might help shed light on choosing an intervention, and developing a plan for sharing or publishing the results of any interventions early in the change process. This allows the advocate to describe a journey in search of the positive core at school and the cultivation of the wellness domain skill-set.

7 Using Relational Dialogues to Nurture Engaged Inquiry

> Thus, in dialogue, each person does not attempt to *make common* certain ideas or items of information that are already known to him [sic]. Rather it may be said that the two people are making something *in common*, i.e., creating something new together.
>
> (David Bohm, 1996, p. 2, italics in original)

In Chapter 7, we explore in greater depth how to take action to enact PIP Phase 2: Engaged Inquiry and AI Phase 2: Relational Dialogue. When considering possibilities, educator advocates build upon the relational connection they have established to initiate dreams about possibilities for collaborative actions. Educator advocates engage in conversations with colleagues and community members and begin to focus possibilities in order to make collaborative decisions about a well-defined action. Engaged inquiry is the stage designed to continue building on Relational Connections to generate conversations about possible actions. Dialogues and engaged inquiry move toward closure on a challenge to be faced, decisions about the best ways to confront the challenge, and actions to address the challenge. The goal is to move conversations, alliances, and collaborative efforts toward action designed to improve the school wellness and learning power outcomes for all students. Thus, taking one or two pathways that build on current assets or possibilities that are constructed anew to address specific challenges in the school.

For researchers and facilitators who want a broad perspective on this process, Chevalier and Buckles (2013) have written a text on participatory action research methodology for engaged inquiry designed for those in voluntary, academic, private, and government sectors. The companion handbook provides "adapted and new tools and processes to engage people and mobilize evidence in complex settings involving multiple stakeholders. They draw inspiration from different disciplines, theoretical perspectives and methodological approaches" (p. 3).

Young and Kaffenberger (2009) offer an overview of ways for helping school counseling professionals make data work to inform change efforts.

Talk with community members, leaders, and colleagues who might serve as allies. Who are individuals with organizational influence who might even be termed key stakeholders? Key stakeholders are those folks, like administrators, who can help or hinder your efforts to bring about change. Key stakeholders are also folks such as secretaries, coaches, and others who are quite capable of speaking positively or negatively about what you are doing or not doing to help students.

Seeing and Hearing Activity 7.1

PIP Phase 2: Engaged Inquiry

PIP Step 4. Using available school-based data, baseline, comparative, and data trends are investigated and reflected upon by the learning community. Student advocates support the learning community in considering: What questions should be posed about the data? And What do we hope to learn? How do we want to lifescape our school?

Reflective PIP Activity: Gather existing data, such as test scores, attendance, etc. Initiate defining surveys to obtain additional data. Ask yourself what questions will bridge the information gaps? For instance: Why are your English learners making progress in mathematics and science, but not in English language/arts?

While gathering data, it is important for educator advocates and administrators to dream about possibilities for lifescaping with diverse community members (teachers, students, other administrators, helping professionals, and families) as much as possible. They can help you as you work to build a collaborative effort to lifescape the school in positive, creative, and inclusive ways. Without their help and alliance change efforts may get stuck at roadblocks and barriers. It is also important to recognize that the site administrators may have pressures from the district superintendent and school board that others in the room do not know about or can be privy to. In order to get to Collaborative Action, it is vital to foster Relational Connections and to dream and imagine fresh possibilities via Engaged Inquiry. This chapter offers tools for deepening Relational Connection and Engaged Inquiry: Mapping the Driving and Restraining Forces (MDRF) Worksheet (see Appendix G), the Core Needs Assessments (CNA) (see Appendix E), and Focus Groups (see Appendix H).

Mapping the Driving and Restraining Forces (MDRF) Worksheet. Mapping the Driving and Restraining Forces (MDRF) Worksheet is a variation using Kurt Lewin's Force Field Analysis and is designed to enable practitioners to assess both organizational context and the personal context supporting and restraining change. Kurt Lewin (1936) was a social psychologist who articulated action research as a method for generating ongoing change in systems; Lewin even gave us the formula that behavior is a dynamic function of persons interacting within their environments: $B = f(P \times E)$ (Conyne & Cook, 2004). Driving forces supporting change are viewed as assets and the forces constraining or restraining change are described as challenges. The MDRF Worksheet template offers a mapping format for laying out an overview of those assets supporting movement toward goals or change and those challenges pulling away from the goal or change. Those forces pulling away from the goal or from any change may simply be the forces of the status quo, such as when members of the school community talk about the students as not being academic, interested in learning, etc. It may be important for the MDRF to be completed by different individuals and different groups. For instance, the site principal may want to complete the MDRF in order to view and understand various pressures from diverse groups, whereas the school counselor team may want to complete the MDRF in order to concentrate the conversation on their evolving school counseling program. The MDRF will vary, depending on who completes it.

One way to use the MDRF Worksheet is to map organizational assets and challenges in order to develop a graphic overview of the situational context in the department or school where change is being initiated. The two key questions guiding the MDRF Worksheet are: 1) What are the assets that are aligned with or promoting change, such as an anti-bullying assembly, in the organization? 2) What are the challenges that are holding change back and, essentially, supporting the status quo, such as limiting anti-bullying efforts to a one-shot school-wide assembly? Mapping the assets and challenges enables participatory leaders in schools to develop a more concrete understanding of the stories told and the data obtained. What and who support change? What and who feel safer with the status quo? The objective is not to judge but to understand the forces, and then learn from individuals supporting the status quo what might help them shift toward ongoing efforts to lifescape your school community.

Another way of using the MDRF Worksheet is to look at individual assets and challenges. Again, there are two key questions. 1) How does this individual embody or endorse assets that are aligned with promoting change in the department? 2) What are the challenges that are holding this individual back from championing change and, essentially, feeling their preferred professional position is to support the status quo. For example, a principal or assistant principal might be very interested in championing certain types of change, only to be constrained by the directives and mandates from those in higher positions within the district. Mapping the MDRF Worksheet in this case allows educator advocates to map those forces so that the pressures of the administrator can be viewed from a different perspective that allows for curiosity and alignment with assets rather than frustration and anger about challenges. The participatory leader is pushed to find out where to begin the conversation. Although advocacy and use of data still might be used to expose how the status quo might be harming students, it is still wise to understand and have compassion for the various pressures that leaders work under in their roles. The point here is to understand, to keep the conversation and story moving, and to define goals in a manner that aligns as much as possible with key stakeholders' assets and understandings.

Mapping the MDRF Worksheet enables student advocates to map driving and restraining forces at the organizational and the personal level. Having such a map enables the advocate to build on assets rather than get bogged down in complaint conversations about the challenges that prevent change or maintain the status quo. Mapping at either level enables practitioners to invite others into conversations that focus on relational possibilities and assets, which are the key to change because the goal is to talk about what we can do together to bring about what might be.

Seeing and Hearing Activity 7.2

Please complete the Mapping the Driving and Restraining Forces Worksheet found in Appendix G. Reflect in writing about what you have mapped. Consider the implications of your responses for the students you serve as a professional.

Seeing and Hearing Activity 7.3

PIP Phase 2: Engaged Inquiry

PIP Step 4. Continue engaged inquiry with the learning community to address the problem or challenge. Additional data are collected from teachers, parents, students, and other community members. Qualitative and quantitative data are gathered through surveys, focus groups, meetings, dialogues, school walk-throughs, and program observations.

Core Needs Assessments (CNA). The second tool is the Core Needs Assessments (CNA), five very short instruments designed as basic needs assessments that target students, teachers, parents, school administrators, and school staff responses regarding the vision and impact (outcomes) of the school counseling and student services program. Although promoting safety and wellness is central to each instrument, these instruments are short and easily adapted for different school contexts. They are referred to as core assessment because they have an essential core across all five needs assessments, not because they have defined a common core that holds for all schools. Each of the assessments does ask one common question about safety, which should be a concern on every campus in the United States.

In adapting and using the CNA for use with students, parents, teachers, administrators, support staff, and the community, it is important to realize that all five data sources do not have to be administered at the same time or when promoting a specific systemic change, even though it is always wonderful to get more data. It is also important to consider how many questions and how much data the research team members want to analyze. Thus, be aware of participant fatigue and be aware of investigator fatigue. Getting half-hearted responses does not help, nor does having piles of unanalyzed data in a drawer. The point is to make the data useful in helping you move toward the changes being conceptualized during the Relational Possibilities stage. Lifescaping is a continuous process that does not have to take place all at the same time.

The CNA can be administered in one period of time, or sequenced over several terms. The CNA depends on the research goals of the participatory leader and research team. If there is a push to move from a school counseling department with no comprehensive program toward becoming a department with a comprehensive program, then getting data from all five instruments would be helpful, as would conversations within the department about various avenues for developing a comprehensive model, such as the *ASCA national model* (2012), Dimmitt et al. (2007), Gysbers and Henderson (2012), Johnson et al. (2006), etc. The point is to think about what data are needed and the best possible sequence for obtaining data.

Additionally, before administering any instrument in a school, check with the school and district policy and provide a consent form to each person. Also, if you are a professional-in-training, check your Human Subjects requirements at your university. The point is ethical, but it is also about being mindfully invitational when asking others for information or their perspective about the impact of the student services program. An example of a generic parent permission form is provided in Appendix F. The example provided was reviewed and approved by the school site, school district, and the Human Subjects Review at the university. Please pay attention to and adapt the permission form for your specific context.

Seeing and Hearing Activity 7.4

Please consult with your supervisor before administering the Core Needs Assessment (see Appendix E). Also, remember to get approval from Human Subjects. The results from this instrument will provide abundant information about the student services on campus.

Focus Groups. Focus groups are powerful tools for promoting informative, reflective, and evolving conversations concentrated on finding out how to improve student learning outcomes, engagement, and participation in school communities (e.g., Ainsworth, 2010; Chappuis et al., 2005; Field & Baker, 2004; Finser, 2007; Harris et al., 2014; Krueger & Casey, 2009; Larson, Grudens-Schuck, & Lundy, 2004; Truebridge, 2014; WestEd, n.d.). In schools, focus groups can empower students, especially if what is shared in the group is used in some way to prompt changes or action toward changes. The importance of focus groups is that they can create space for sharing untold stories, and define safe space where truth can be spoken to power without fear of repercussions or retributions. Focus groups in this text are not about venting but about opening dialogical space to find the narratives undergirding any frustration or anger and moving toward the positive core—what we are referring to as relational possibilities. Focus groups can foster a composing space where new relational possibilities can be generated and defined to build and revise the stories being lived.

Seeing and Hearing Activity 7.5

Focus groups provide abundant useful information. See Appendix H. Please follow the guidelines for initiating focus groups and the ethical implications inherent in conducting such groups, including the safety and well-being of all participants. If you lack experience leading focus groups, it is important to conduct the focus group with someone with experience.

There are numerous types of focus groups, ranging from those concerned with marketing products (see David Foster Wallace's (2004) short story "Mr. Squishy" as an horrific example) to those attempting to give voice to all members of communities. This chapter will be limited to describing three types of focus groups: a focus story group, a fishbowl story group, and a video story focus group. Each type offers a practical focus group approach that can be used in schools to extend and deepen conversations about relational possibilities (see Appendix H for Focus Group, Fishbowl Story Group, and Video Story Focus Group Guidelines and support materials).

The focus story group allows for gathering information and narratives from select groups run by a facilitator. The focus story groups foster a reflective space where new relational possibilities can be generated and defined by those participating in the focus group. The members generate the core conversation based on a series of prompts, and they are encouraged to move toward defining at least one specific action as a focus group outcome. The essential question for those participating in the focus group approach shared in this text is: What can be done to make this a more connected school community that promotes the wellness and learning power of all students?

The fishbowl story focus group engages in a similar format run by a facilitator, only the six to eight-member focus group is surrounded by adults or invited observers who remain silent, listening to and bearing witness to what is being said by the members of the focus group. The essential difference between a focus story group and a fishbowl focus group is that the fishbowl has a group of adults or observers sitting outside of the group bearing witness to what is being said. The process places the adults in a position where they listen and bear witness to what is important to students, and the students experience greater validation and power as they speak their own truth to the adults who are showing the willingness to listen.

Core questions in the back of the facilitator's mind include:

• What are our strengths?
• How are others demonstrating their belief in students?
• What have adults done to effectively show care, support, and belief in the learning power of students in this school?
• Where/when do we struggle? Why?
• What are some possible directions we could take to promote student wellness and success?
• What is one small step we can take together, shoulder to shoulder, as adults and students?
• What is our plan for the first step?

The video story focus group comes into play when adults cannot "find time" to participate in the fishbowl group. In this case, the focus group can be recorded and edited by the focus group leader and the students into a coherent message for adults. The use of recordings involves permissions and Human Subjects, but more importantly, the leader must focus on the positive core and sharing the most powerful elements of the session that inform the future forming aspirations of the students.

Engaged Inquiry

Engaged inquiry involves entering into conversations with different members of the school community in ways that focus on promoting the wellness of students and the rest of the community. Although aligned with efforts to develop comprehensive school counseling programs, this text recognizes that ecological counselors trying to promote relational wellness and learning power in the schools are going to be in settings where there are pressing concerns that seem to be far away from developing a comprehensive school counseling program. As mentioned above, school community challenges include conflict, violence, bullying, truancy, graffiti, and lack of engagement on campus. Schools without clear comprehensive programs may easily frame interventions and specific results-based efforts in terms of movement toward more comprehensive student support programs. In other words, relational dialogues with school community stakeholders move toward defining interventions and programs in terms of the development of comprehensive school support programs.

Through engaged inquiry ideas are put on the table, discussed, and explored in ways that might breathe life into them by those who are willing to move toward action. This is the stage that involves imagination and dreaming, as well as the beginning steps toward narrowing down the decision to talking about the first step. What is to be done? Through engaged inquiry challenges and problems are deeply examined from multiple perspectives in order to generate possible actions designed to lifescape the school in more inclusive and strength-building ways. Table 7.1 provides examples of problems and challenges as well as possible actions to address the underlying issues.

Table 7.1 Problems/Challenges and Possible Actions

Problem/Challenge	Possible Action
Conflict, violence, and bullying on campus—Perception: Lack care and support	Making Peace program focused on personal/social competence
Under-represented youth not meeting college eligibility index—Perception: Lack of high expectations for all students	PUENTE and/or AVID programs building sense of learning power
High ninth grade failure rate—Perception: Lack of connectedness and learning power	Transition and academic support program that helps develop decision making skills
Truancy, graffiti, lack of student engagement—Perception: Lack of opportunities for meaningful participation and contribution	Opportunities for contributions and developing a sense of purpose at school

Engaged inquiry moves toward loose and dreamy openness geared toward encouraging multiple perspectives about possible solutions, whereas the collaborative action narrows down possibilities and makes commitment to focused actions that will be taken and assessed based on the outcomes they bring. Thus, relational dialogues is about generating ideas and possibilities, whereas relational action is about deciding what focused action can be done together to promote more wellness as measured by academic, personal/social, career learning, and contributions to the school/ community.

While exploring relational dialogues, recognize that there are numerous programs and interventions reviewed and discussed in Galassi and Akos (2007), a book that should be in every student advocate's library. Those interested in generating conversations focused on school program development should refer to that resource and other core resources concerned with developing school counseling programs, such as the ASCA *national model* (2012), Gysbers and Henderson (2012), Hatch (2014), Johnson et al. (2006), Squier et al. (2014), etc. Simply stated, get those classics and refer to them when engaging in relational dialogues and moving toward collaborative actions that involve steps toward program development. Having program development in mind when embracing an ecological perspective and relational dialogues is helpful because school support programs are best when guided by result-based practices and concern for agreed-upon student outcomes. Engaged inquiry moves from talking about what is and what might be toward taking meaningful, measurable, and realistic action. Relational actions move toward defining what student advocates will do in the school and assessing the results in terms of outcomes for all students. Those outcomes usually focus on personal/social, academic, and career learning, as well as contributions to the school and greater community. Thus, in many ways, relational dialogues are partly about engaging the learning community in conversations and then moving those conversations toward actions that will change the world and experience of students.

In order to achieve movement from engaged inquiry to collaborative actions, it is vital to have allies, advocates, colleagues, friends, and school community stakeholders who are willing to enter into the conversations, look at the data, dream about the possibilities, and move toward actions. Otherwise, there is a chance that the process will get bogged down in conversations, where there is a lot of "We should . . ." with very little movement toward thoughtful action directed toward outcomes that are assessed, revised, and acted upon again. At the very least, engaged inquiry requires a commitment to joining with others to do one thing differently and to assess the results. Even if it is a small step, it is important to move engaged inquiry toward collaborative action.

Promoting relational wellness ecologically means responding to the learning needs within the school community and insuring that members experience school as a series of life-enhancing practices, regardless of how well-developed and defined the comprehensive school counseling program is. Conversations and dialogues about promoting wellness can move in myriad directions. To move toward collaborative actions, it is important to be able to talk about possible pathways. Besides those texts linked directly to developing comprehensive school counseling programs, engaged inquiry opens up opportunities to enact different approaches. For instance, Winslade and Williams (2012), Williams and Brown (2012), and Goleman et al. (2012) provide interventions and programs that can inform student advocates in how they can collaborate with the entire school community to promote learning power and relational wellness in their schools. Each approach describes interventions and programs that can be tested and assessed in practice. Each is shared here as an example illustrating how engaged inquiry can lead to collaborative actions that influence the entire school community. Again, although each could be aligned with comprehensive school counseling efforts, each could be used as a springboard and first step toward constructing a school counseling program or gaining support for new student services, such as tutoring, volunteer programs, etc. These are merely examples of what might be put forward during engaged inquiry to determine collaborative actions that are assessed for their efficacy. The key point is answering the question: What is one thing we can do to improve the challenge we have defined?

Winslade and Williams (2012) present a narrative and restorative justice approach to developing safe and peaceful schools in order to address school community challenges such as conflict, violence, bullying, and truancy. The authors begin by recognizing that conflict is inevitable, and then go on to offer counselors, administrators, and teachers tools for helping to construct peaceful interactions in school. The authors offer a narrative perspective in how to promote peace at schools. Interventions range from specific counseling techniques to mediation, peer mediation, restorative conferencing and practices, circle conversations, undercover anti-bullying teams, and guidance lessons. Although the approach could guide a comprehensive narrative relational decision, any one of the interventions could be the foundation of a more focused first step, too.

Williams and Brown (2012) propose a program for integrating gardening into the entire curriculum and school community. Although the authors do not talk about a role for student advocates in the schools, the approach they offer could guide relational dialogues led by helping professionals to address lack of engagement on campus. The key point here is that schools integrating gardens and place into their curriculum connects students to a greater sense of community (Smith & Williams, 1999; Sobel, 2004; Stone, 2009; Williams & Brown, 2012). By promoting relational dialogues that integrate gardening into the curriculum, student advocates begin to explore ways to connect students to school as a learning place, both inside and outside the classroom. Martin Luther King Junior Middle School in Berkeley, California has an edible garden program where students work in the garden and learn about the soil, biology, ecology, and nutrition in relation to the garden. Teachers and students are excited about the content. School counselors walk and talk with kids in the gardens as a way of calming down and getting grounded.

At a deeper level, the edible garden bridges the chasm between high-status and low-status knowledge. High-status knowledge is abstract, in-the-head theoretical, decontextualized, and associated with university education, whereas low-status knowledge is concrete, manual, craft, contextualized, and associated with vocational training (Bowers, 2000; Williams & Brown, 2012). High-status knowledge is privileged and craft knowledge and vocational arts in the United States have been marginalized over the past thirty years. The notion of gardening in schools can be viewed as an antiquated but quaint nostalgic desire to bring back a lost past, rather than a deep cultural expression of connection to the earth and living systems. Gardening is a practical craft that is learned over time where lessons are frequently learned one season at a time. Gardening is also a craft where the learner is mentored in participatory action that is concerned with living soils, nurturing plants, and resulting flavors.

Goleman et al. (2012) provide case studies, stories, and approaches for engaging colleagues and communities in cultivating eco-literate learning communities. For student advocates, their notion of learning circles is a powerful way to invite conversation and dialogue about learning, community, and integration into the ecosystem where all are connected. The format is similar to forming any group, but there is much effort to connect to the greater community and the physical space where the group meets. Winslade and Williams (2012), Williams and Brown (2012), and Goleman et al. (2012) illustrate how conversations and relational dialogues can lead to important decisions about interventions and programs, as well as significant discussions about the purpose of education.

Advocacy and Participatory Leadership

In order to initiate Phase 2 of the PIP or AI, participatory leaders are advised to reflect on the four skill-sets described in the wellness domain: performative focus, vital engagement, self-reflectiveness, and relational connectedness. All four skill-sets are necessary to be successful in Phase 2 of PIP and AI. Performative focus calls for personal and social competence in asking more difficult questions. Vital engagement calls for being excited about the prospect of doing something to address even one small problem. Self-reflectiveness opens advocates to listening to critical questions without personalizing them; that is, being grounded with equanimity. Finally, relational connectedness is needed to maintain positive working relationships even when subjecting the work to critical questions.

It is important for participatory leaders to know how to move from PIP Engaged Inquiry and AI Relational Dialogue toward PIP Collaborative Action and AI Relational Action, which involve carrying out what is decided upon by those collaborating on the project. Participatory leaders work to deepen conversations, gather more information, and move their allies toward defining a challenge to be addressed. Using the tools provided in this chapter will help leaders move the conversation, inquiry, and dialogue forward. The question becomes what tool do we choose to use at this point in time. The leader does not have to use all the tools, and might want to be selective in choosing one that will help the most in the present moment and circumstances.

Chapter Summary

This chapter provides a number of tools for moving from PIP Initiating Conversations and Identifying Challenges or building AI Relational Connections toward PIP Engaged Inquiry and AI Relational Dialogue. The move to more critical questioning involves equanimity and begins by using tools such as the Mapping Driving and Restraining Forces (MDRF) to explore the forces that would hinder or support change efforts. The MDRF should be used by individuals, such as site principals, and groups, such as school counselor teams, in order to assess the driving and restraining forces for change from their own professional perspectives before they use the MDRF in larger groups. Core Needs Assessments provide survey information from multiple perspectives, as well. The Core Needs Assessment versions provided may be adapted to fit the unique needs of a variety of sites and communities. Focus groups are a powerful approach for drilling down with a small group in order to develop a deeper story about an issue or concern. The focus group leader should be an advocate who is viewed as neutral, and not an authority figure such as a site administrator. School counselors, school psychologists, and school social workers are generally trained in conducting groups and should be competent in leading focus story groups. Engaged inquiry involves interrogating data and stories in a manner that subjects the data and stories to critical question with the intention to bring out workable plans for action. Gaps and blind spots are considered as challenges to be addressed, defined, explored, and confronted—not denied. The essential goal becomes: What is one thing we can do to address the challenge before us or to lifescape the learning community we desire?

8 Pursuing Relational, Collaborative Action

> That we accept the world as it is does not in any sense weaken our desire
> to change it into what we believe it should be—it is necessary to begin
> where the world is if we are going to change it to what we think it should
> be. That means working in the system.
>
> (Saul Alinsky, 1971, p. xix)

In Chapter 8, we explore in greater depth how to take action to enact
PIP Phase 3: Collaborative Action and AI Phase 3: Relational Action.
Collaborative action and relational action are both about making choices,
asking questions, taking responsibility, making commitments with others
in lifescaping the school and community where you are. Recognizing what
is should not diminish future forming and lifescaping actions. Choices
involve joining with others to collaborate in a process that involves
answering key questions generated in the data, and fostering conversations
that point toward taking action after the relational connections and engaged
inquiry phase. For instance, after reviewing the data in an engaged inquiry
about a school-wide concern, two core questions are developed: "What
can we do together to improve the number of African-American students
meeting the college eligibility index at our school?" and "What actions
have been taken or can we take to compose new stories about how our
department helps African-American, economically disadvantaged kids, and
other under-represented kids succeed?" Core questions and concerns range
from academic concerns just mentioned to personal, social, career, school
connectedness, etc. The key points are: first, defining the lifescape we want
to create or the challenge being addressed collectively;s and second, what
has been done in the past to address the challenge or lifescape the school
community? In terms of the second point, it is important to find out what,
if anything, has worked in the past, even if it was successful for a short
duration or in some small way. Being curious and using mindful
wonderment regarding what worked is an important way to respect past
efforts and to invite allies or become allies with leaders of those past efforts.
Most importantly, what are the students and their families saying about
what did and didn't work in the past and what is and isn't working now?

Collaborative action moves conversations from dreaming about lifescaping possibilities of what might be and if only . . . into clear, concrete, specific, and measurable goal(s) that are framed in terms of time limits, meaningfulness, obtainability, and analysis of the impact of the actions taken on the school system. Collaborative actions require commitment. What is my responsibility? Who else is making a commitment? What is the first well-defined step in the change process? How do we keep the change process going? How can specific actions be defined in a way that enables measurement and evaluation of the progress? How do we continue to engage students in the assessment of what is and isn't working? Goals, timelines, and responsibilities are defined. Dialogues shift to inviting collaborations, allies, and friends to commit to specific responsibilities in acting or supporting the meaningful goal. The ASCA (2012) offers a SMART Goals Worksheet that can be quite useful for defining goals; SMART stands for Specific, Measurable, Action-Oriented, Realistic, and Timely. Our concern is that SMART can drift toward pure instrumentalism because it has no meaning or insurance of vital and participatory engagement, which from our perspective is a problematic. As a modest alternative, the PIP and AI Action Worksheet (Appendix I) is designed to assist individuals and teams in decision making that moves toward reflective and relational actions. The PIP and AI Action Worksheet helps to define a decision making process with specific goal(s), measures, time constraints, and analysis of action. The worksheet explores the meaningfulness of the action to stakeholders, how realistic the action seems, and how the actions are aligned with current stories in the ecosystem. In short, the PIP and AI Action Worksheet is a tool to guide decisions about the actions practitioners and their allies can choose to take in achieving meaningful goals defined in the collaborative process. As part of considering the ecological and relational context, the PIP and AI Action Worksheet has one section that concentrates on exploring the meaningfulness of the goal to possible allies and one section that centers on how the goals and actions might be aligned with the values and interests embedded in the stories shared by other stakeholders. It should be said that both the SMART and PIP and AI Action Worksheets are tools, and practitioners are advised to use the one that works best for them to achieve their ends.

Action Activity 8.1

Please complete the PIP and AI Action Worksheet in Appendix I. Read the text below before you begin the process. The object is to make a decision about how you and others are going to use professional time and resources.

First, it is vital to define a goal(s) that is clear, concrete, specific, and measurable that has support from key stakeholders; it is also vital to be flexible to the context, situation, and circumstances that arise in the moment. Define the goal as something that can be seen in terms of data and develop a step-by-step pathway for getting there. Be able to measure distance from and to the goal concretely, such as the percentage of under-represented youth (African-American and Latino) in the school that meet the college eligibility index. As an example, say the current percentage of African-American and Latino students meeting the college eligibility index at the time of graduation is 12 percent. The learning community agrees that the goal is to raise that number by 3 percent to 15 percent in one year, and then to 45 percent of graduates within 3 years as a result of a college-going culture program that is being implemented. The goal is clear, concrete, specific, and measureable. If there are unforeseen obstacles, the three-year goal can be revised, but goals are still defined in terms of short term and long term.

Second, as shown above, frequently goals will determine measures. In the case above the percentage of under-represented students meeting the college eligibility index is the measure. The current 12 percent data would be the baseline, or starting point, for measuring progress; the aspirational goal might be to get 100 percent of students to meet the index, but knowing where you are helps clarify realistic goals to mark your way toward the long-term goal. The first annual goal could be 15 percent, the three-year goal could be 45 percent, and the aspirational goal would always be 100 percent. Questions about where the eligibility index data come from would have to be clarified. Is this self-report? Does the school data system track college eligibility index data? Can college eligibility index data be disaggregated by gender, race, and ethnic group? In other words, even if the goal and measures have been decided, it is important to determine how practical and realistic it is to track the data. It may be necessary to advocate for tracking certain data just to get the conversation going. Obviously, the first goal might be to define ways for tracking important data at the site level. Recognizing the limitations in how data are collected is a continuous challenge and the problem is clearly evident in the various ways schools and districts track dropout data (Vernez, 2008). In fact, without adequate data, the collaborative action might begin with advocacy in demanding forms of data that can be tracked to determine the quality of education being offered to all students (Holcomb-McCoy, 2007; House & Martin, 1998; Lee, 2007; Miller & Garran, 2008).

Third, there are only so many things that can be done in a day. It is important to make sure enough time has been budgeted to achieve the defined goal. What are the other demands on the advocate's time? Will advocates be stretched and accomplish the goal or make commitments they cannot keep? This is where those who do the minimum choose to do the minimum and where those who are oriented to stretch themselves, do just that. Professionals have to judge what is minimum and what is going to cause undue stress or even put them in a position where they cannot keep their commitments. Practitioners must choose what is going to help them best to grow as professionals; this is what relational decisions are about, maintaining effective relationships with others, defining responsibilities, and staying vibrant and on the growing edge. A collaborative action is defined by community engagement in addressing a challenge, not by a single individual's heroic efforts to save the world.

Fourth, it is important to explore how possible allies think about the goals being shaped and defined. School helping professionals' colleagues, counselors, psychologists, social workers, and community mental health workers are important sources of support and feedback, as are students, teachers, administrators, parents, and other stakeholders. The PIP and AI Action Worksheet is designed to move toward collaborative actions by educator advocates to consider and talk about what is most important. The essential point here is to determine whom the allies and change supporters are and define the goal together. Find out how important each community member thinks the goal is and how they will support efforts to achieve the goal(s).

Fifth, the PIP and AI Action Worksheet offers a quick way to assess how realistic the goal is in terms of time frame and in terms of attainment in relationship with others. Assessing and mapping the driving and restraining forces is one of the steps to determining the systemic barriers and supports to reaching the goal(s), including time budgeted for project, time requested from allies and other stakeholders. Because collaborative actions result from ongoing conversations with those involved, this is the stage where some goals are broken down into smaller goals. For instance, maybe there is a desire to build a comprehensive school counseling program based on Gysbers and Henderson (2012) or the *ASCA national model* (2012), but there is little enthusiasm from colleagues or support from the school administration. A collaborative action would not be made to push for a full embrace of a comprehensive program, but a collaborative action could be to take one step by conducting a program audit, or some other action might bring more colleagues into the conversation about the need for a comprehensive program. Collaborative actions can become baby steps toward larger goals. Collaborative actions are important because they build relationships within the organization in order to increase the capacity to move toward goals that enhance student wellness that are assessed and shared.

Collaborative action frequently comes into play due to unforeseen conversations in the school ecosystem. Perhaps the superintendent and school board are talking about cutting back on the school counseling program because they are not sure what school counselors and other student support personnel do to help students get into college. Conceivably, the school counselors could take collaborative action after their own possibilities conversations lead them to track data to show how counselors help students meet the college eligibility index. The index data they track would be most illustrative if it provides outcome data that show what counselors did to teach and orient more students to strive for and meet the eligibility index, rather than merely sharing process data that showed the number of students who attended guidance activities that focused on the eligibility index (see ASCA, 2012).

Embraced as a first step, tracking such outcome data about what was done to help students would help move colleagues forward toward sharing ongoing actions to help students increase their academic achievement. Collaborative action in the AI process is geared toward taking active steps; they are also relational, rather than mechanical. Collaborative action is part of a relational process directed toward nurturing learning power and wellness in all students. In this example, such a step would have to include informing the superintendent and school board about the impact these advocates have upon students trying to get into college.

Sixth, the PIP and AI Action Worksheet affirms how important it is to analyze the impact of actions taken. Chapter 9 (Community Assessment and Reflection) will discuss the importance of analyzing and assessing the impact of the actions taken. It is important to analyze the impact of the actions taken. The PIP and AI Action Worksheet enables those involved with the participatory inquiry process to connect collaborative actions to community assessment and reflection. when taking action, it is important to consider how to assess the impact of those actions.

Seventh, collaborative action is central to the PIP and AI Action Worksheet, and it is vital to assist practitioners in wondering about and reflecting upon how their values, hopes, dreams, and stories are aligned with those expressed in small and large ways in the community ecosystem. Collaborative actions are about honoring what is best within other individuals, and the aspirational, life-enhancing stories shared in the school, district, and community. Linking actions with an understanding of what is best and most life-enhancing in the community is an attempt to find ground where respect and care for the community and its children can be talked about in a forthright manner. Taking such a position requires helpers to act like anthropologists who listen deeply to what is best in the culture and community and to act as advocates who are willing to take positions on behalf of students' wellness and what is best in the community. This also means acting as advocates who are willing to take positions on behalf of the most marginalized students' wellness and what is best in helping them to become recognized as integral parts of the community. Listening deeply and observing systemic actions critically is essential to examining unexamined assumptions that may be hindering student growth, present and future well-being (i.e., access to STEAM pathways).

After reviewing the completed PIP and AI Action Worksheet, individuals or working groups should be able to move forward to take informed collaborative action—defining the goal(s) more precisely, choosing an intervention or program that will help move toward the goal(s), and selecting a method for evaluating and sharing progress made toward achieving the goal. This is the stage where working groups decide upon the challenges to be addressed and the specific actions to address those challenges. The choice may be to conduct a program audit and take a step toward constructing a comprehensive school counseling program. The choice could be to embrace some aspect or the entire narrative approach to promoting peaceful schools, as Winslade and Williams (2012) offer, or even some aspect of Williams and Brown's (2012) school garden approach to education. Essentially, the action-taking process enables choices to be made and goals to be defined.

Deepening the Literature Review and Taking Action

Using your initial literature review, focus your attention on your topic. Research articles, books, websites, and related materials that have investigated or intervened on the challenge being addressed. Define your audience. Is it your community of practice working group? Other allies? Your site administrator? The superintendent? The school board? Your professor? Sharpen your literature review to speak to the audience you are choosing. You want to show evidence and generate a narrative that speaks to how that challenge has been addressed in order to present how and what you want to do to address the challenge in your local and specific school.

Action Activity 8.2

Phase 2: Engaged Inquiry

PIP Step 4. Using professional texts and library resources, responses to the problem are researched in the professional literature. Resources within the school community are assessed and reflected on in framing how to address the challenge.

PIP Activity: Use internet, professional, and library resources to find what works best to address the challenge.

Share your literature review with your colleagues, your community of practice, your learning community, and others working with you on the project.

Action Activity 8.3

Phase 3: Collaborative Action

PIP Step 5. The problem is defined and shared by the learning community and a strategy to address the issue is proposed.

PIP Activity: Review the PIP and AI Action Worksheet in Appendix I; describe what you have committed to, even if it is one small step.

After sharing your defined lifescaping vision, problem, and strategy being considered with your working group and making any necessary adjustments, you are ready to take action. Review the PIP and AI Action Worksheet and take action. Think do-it-yourself or consider the French term *bricolage*, which means to tinker or improvise as you are doing something. Be informed by bricolage and the need to adjust and shift from the ideas on paper, in your head, and in your conversations to the actual situation and context where you take action. Makeshift adjustments in action research are perfectly normal. Pay attention to and document your bricolage responses. Think in terms of the PIP and the AI process; sometimes it is one step backwards and two steps forward. You are learning a new skill and way of being in action; be patient and forgiving of yourself. Look with equanimity rather than negative judgment on your work and efforts. Beginners frequently become overly self-critical at times when they need abundant self-compassion.

Reflective Moment 8.1

As you consider possible actions to address the identified problem/challenge, ask:

- Who is participating? Who is responsible for what?
- How do we define this support effort?
- What are we (am I) going to do? What are our goal(s)?
- What is the first step we/I will take?
- How will we know if we are successful? What measures will be used?
- How will we assess and share our results?

The next chapter looks more closely at methods and approaches for assessing and documenting progress toward goals defined during the action-taking process.

Advocacy and Participatory Leadership

Participatory leaders are cheerleaders and innovators during AI Phase 3: Relational Action and PIP Phase 3: Collaborative Action. In order to initiate Phase 3 of the PIP or AI, participatory leaders are advised to reflect on the four skill-sets described in the wellness domain: performative focus, vital engagement, self-reflectiveness, and relational connectedness. Performative focus calls for personal and social competence in taking decisive action.

Vital engagement calls for being excited about the prospect of taking action to address even one small problem. Self-reflectiveness opens advocates to bricolage and makeshift adjustments that will be necessary when the action begins. Finally, relational connectedness maintains positive working relationships and communication during the entire project.

The PIP and AI Action Worksheet can help inform and guide the action by enabling review, adjustment, and movement in the action. Participatory leaders recognize that what is worked out on paper and in one's head have to be adjusted to the circumstances in the school on the day the action begins. Participatory leaders embrace equanimity when viewing the action. Successes and obstacles both inform the pathway of the project. Expectations are concentrated on bricolage and day-to-day successful working and the ability to step back before pressing the project forward.

Chapter Summary

This chapter concentrates on the movement toward action. Both PIP Phase 3: Collaborative Action and AI Phase 3: Relational Action highlight pathways to successful action. The chapter shares the PIP and AI Action Worksheet, which enables the advocate to summarize each PIP and AI phase in a manner that allows for a reflective action-oriented process that is connected to bricolage and the need to adjust to the lived reality in the school when the action is taking place. The Action Activity boxes in this chapter are designed to keep the work moving and alive. Action implies movement and life, as well as the need to reflect upon any actions taken.

9 Practicing Relational, Community Assessment and Reflection

> Research is an endless, methodical quest with provisional and inconclusive results, because all things more or less hang together: relationism, not relativism.
>
> (Arne Naess, 2002, p. 4)

In Chapter 9, we explore in greater depth how to take action to enact PIP Phase 4: Community Assessment and Reflection and AI Phase 4: Relational Assessment. Collaborative actions are intimately connected to and ultimately define community assessment and reflection.

Reflective Moment 9.1

Phase 3: Collaborative Action

Step 6. Actions are taken to put the agreed upon strategy(s) into practice

PIP Activity: Be mindful of your actions.

- What happened?
- What did we learn? What worked? Why?
- What could be improved? How?
- What recommendations, adjustments or future action do we recommend?
- Next steps?
- Where are we going?
- What do we still need to know?
- How do we celebrate?

Action/assessment are linked by a slash because results-based practice requires that actions be assessed to determine the impact upon students' lives, learning power, and wellness. Consequences, outcomes, workability, and considerations for what works are keys to decisions about how to proceed. Do the students have more knowledge and skills, or healthier attitudes? Community assessment and reflection inform progressions of ethical action, assessment, and maintaining the story as a living creative act. The community assessment and reflection phase focuses on research as a creative composing process where actions in school systems are viewed as living works-in-progress. The goal is improving results, and not judgmental evaluation.

What are the goal(s) that we are going to act upon in the given time frame? Who are those collaborating with us? What student population are we working with? How well are we engaging and involving the students? Are we inviting students to actively participate in defining the goals or to understand why such goals are being defined? What are our roles and duties? Who is responsible for what? What are we (am I) going to do? What is the first step I will take? How will we know if we are successful? What is the story we will tell?

Still, stories shared are post hoc, after the fact; the stories told in documents, testimonials, and elsewhere do exist in time and space, but they are looking back at the events and making choices about what to tell. Those who construct narratives tell and retell those stories with some or no change as they tell and retell the story, forgetting this or embellishing on that. The document is written, the story is told to the board, the press, parents, etc. Yet, in school systems, a living creative active process must continue if the relational flow and action is going to remain vital. Lifescaping never ends; the issue becomes sustaining what is beautiful and working, while planting something that will enhance the lifescape. Community assessment and reflection is concerned with keeping narratives in motion and using ongoing feedback to nurture the evolution and development of living, never-ending stories. The written document, the story told to the board, the press, parents, and others is merely a marker indicating actions and results in promoting the learning power and relational wellness of all students. In other words, the community assessment and reflection process is about story development in progress. Community assessment and reflection keeps change efforts rolling by documenting the step or steps showing what is being done differently in the moment and what might be improved next. Where are we in relation to the goal? What is different? What has improved? What went well? Such questions mean seeking feedback and assessing clear, specific, and concrete goals. They also mean a continuing conversation about the learning power and relational wellness fostered in school communities. How does the school foster students' learning power and relational wellness? Does the school assess personal/social competence, relational wellness, learning power, or students' sense of purpose at school? What steps are being taken to teach these skills?

The change process should be documented and shared with community members and other interested parties via papers, presentations, postings, or other venues. What was our lifescaping dream? What was our lifescaping image? What happened? These are important questions in both PIP and AI as developmental processes. Celebrate the learning power and wellness brought forth in the effort. Besides mere data, documentation includes reflection and recommendations for next steps. Change is not about waving a magic wand but patient and persistent efforts to bring about fresh stories about learning power and relational wellness in the school community.

Reflective Moment 9.2

Mindfully reflect in writing in response to key questions including:

- What happened?
- What did students learn?
- What future actions should be recommended? Next steps?
- Where are we going from where we are?
- How are positive outcomes celebrated?
- How are negligible or poor outcomes redirected toward achievable goals?

Assessing academic, personal–social (belongingness, connectedness, etc.), graduation, college admission, and other student outcomes is vital when undertaking any action. Any gold standard for assessing school counseling program outcomes would certainly have a taproot in Gysbers and Henderson (2012) and their key text in developing and managing comprehensive school counseling programs. Equally, Johnson et al.'s (2006) results-based, ASCA's (2012) standards-based, Dimmitt et al.'s (2006) evidence-based, Squier et al.'s (2014) construct-based, and the Education Trust's (2000) data-driven approaches are all concerned with student outcomes in school counseling programs. This text in your hand embraces some of the elements from each of these, but like Galassi and Akos (2007), there is emphasis on the promotion of strengths (learning power and relational wellness) as an ongoing process. In the case of this text, it is a future forming, lifescaping process that concentrates on building upon strengths rather than merely upon reducing deficits. In fact, what is done at this phase might be defined as action/assessment, where both action and assessment are tied together to inform what to continue or build upon in the next steps. Action/assessment should be concentrated on finding the best practices at specific school sites for promoting positive youth development, as measured in terms of the actual students' personal/social competence, decision making skills, learning power, and sense of purpose in what they are actually doing at school and in their community.

Thus, assessment should be contextualized in the community ecosystem. Assessment should not be determined based on decontextualized standards that are external to the community or standards that are somehow isolated from the day-to-day experiences of the students being assessed. The PIP and 4-R process are about contextualizing positive youth development and moving school communities toward embracing youth as resources. The PIP and 4-R process help create, define, and build interventions or program components in an effort to foster comprehensive programs as living projects that target student learning power and relational wellness as measured by personal–social competencies, decision making skills, learning power, and students' sense of purpose in what they are doing at school and in their community.

Even if the project has numerous challenges and only gets part way toward the defined goal in the delineated time frame, there is a lesson that should be documented in order to help move the program forward. Even project failures are opportunities to reflect and learn; the point is not condemnation or shame, but learning, growth, and development when attempting to lifescape school communities.

Reflective Moment 9.3

Analyzing the impact of the actions amounts to mapping the steps taken and the outcomes toward achieving the goal(s). Please respond to the following questions:

- What supported reaching the goal and what hindered reaching the goal? How do you know? What might be done differently to improve progress?
- What was done that seemed to have the most impact in moving toward the goal(s)?
- Who were allies in helping move forward?
- Who should be thanked, encouraged, etc.?
- Who should know more about this?
- What's next?

Assessing Actions

The first question driving assessment of action is: How has the students' learning power or relational wellness been enhanced by the program, lessons, interventions, and/or actions taken? Everything else follows that key question. How will we know whether we have moved toward or away from our goal? Can we say that one thing is made better by the actions?

As shown in the first 4-R phases, the positive core is explored, data are accumulated, specific challenges defined, decisions made, and goals defined. Such goals may include increasing the number of under-represented students who meet the college eligibility index, promoting peace by reducing bullying on campus, etc. The crucial point is connecting the goal to be assessed to lessons, interventions, and programs developed to achieve the goal.

Reflective Moment 9.4

At this stage the community is trying to determine how students' personal/social competencies, decision making, learning power, or sense of purpose have been enhanced by the collaborative actions? How do you know? What evidence can you share with skeptical others? Please reflect in writing in response to the following questions.

- What *personal–social competencies* have been taught, modeled, and assessed?
- What *decision making skills* have been taught, modeled, and assessed?
- How has each student's sense of learning power been enhanced? How has their *learning power* been translated into improved grades or academic performance?
- How have the lessons, interventions, and program interventions deepened students' *sense of purpose* in what they are doing at school and in their community?
- What do students have to say about their experiences?

Deciding on what to assess is vital. Thoughtful assessment enables you to say why you know what you know. Grades, attendance, and other such variables may be used in assessing the impact of what is done to help enhance student learning power and relational wellness. Improved grades and number of students meeting the college eligibility index are important measures. At the same time, both what is assessed and the assessment instruments must take into account community context and socially responsible assessment in counseling (Loesch, 2007). In developing a school community beyond the standardized measures used to assess academic performance in schools, it is important to advocate for and to assess students' personal–social competencies, decision making skills, learning power, and sense of purpose in what they are doing at school and in their community. The problem is that there are not always inexpensive, easy-to-use instruments to assess knowledge, skills, and attitudes associated with positive youth development. Results-based practices advocate using rubrics and self-evaluation based on pre-established, expected results. Having students keep electronic learning logs or developing electronic portfolios is another way to track individual and group development (Wakimoto & Lewis, 2014). Defining action research as a school counseling intervention and assessment tool may invite greater collaboration with all community members, including students (Reason & Bradbury, 2008; Reason & Hawkins, 1988; Rowell, 2005, 2006; Stringer, 2014; Whiston, 1996). The PIP and the 4-R process are essentially steps that invite participatory inquiry in the assessment process; sort of a shoulder-to-shoulder invitation to all stakeholders, asserting we can move this school and community forward together in a respectful way.

Sharing the Work

In California, there are a variety of efforts that provide tools for student advocates in the schools to take realistic steps to move their programs forward and for sharing their stories with larger audiences. Two such examples are: 1) The Center for Excellence in School Counseling and Leadership (CESCaL) offers steps for creating Flashlights; and 2) Action Research in School Counseling (www.schoolcounselor-advocate.com/) offers support for generating school counseling action research. A third example is the Social Publishers Foundation (www.socialpublishers foundation.org/) which offers resources to crowd source funding, develops action research, and publishes results. A fourth example from California involves a collaborative effort that started at the Los Angeles Office of Education and the California Department of Education; the Support Personnel Accountability Report Card (SPARC) is a document that can be used for showing how support personnel help all students in the personal/ social, academic, and career domains. In the case of SPARC, it is a first step that can show how the student support program helps students in each of the three domains. The point is that CESCaL, Action Research in School Counseling, Social Publishers Foundation, and SPARC offer tools for advocates to define and assess progress toward achieving measurable goals. These are only four examples; as mentioned earlier, there are additional resources for moving a school counseling program forward such as MEASURE and RAMP.

There are also open-access publications, such as those coming out of the Taos Institute as WorldShare Books (www.taosinstitute.net/worldshare-books). In *Exceeding expectations: An anthology of appreciative inquiry stories in education from around the world*, Dole et al. (2014) offer a very innovative approach to sharing how appreciative inquiry impacts education throughout the world. Their concrete and specific examples from around the world provide a model for sharing PIP and AI projects as well. The point here is that sharing lifescaping and future forming efforts is a way to bring about the world we want to live in or leave for our children and their children.

Sharing results with the school, the district, the board, and the larger community is important to the iterative process of school improvement. One of the concerns we have with the *ASCA national model* (2012) is that it makes only passing mention of action research and how it can be used to promote program development and student success. The current *ASCA national model* edition endorses their approved RAMP and tools ASCA markets. There is not enough conversation and resources regarding diverse approaches for developing school counseling programs, such as action research, SPARC, Flashlight and other pathways. School counselors and other student advocates in the schools need tools they can use in collaboration with each other and other professionals to promote the learning power and wellness of students. What works best may vary depending on context and challenges being addressed; advocates need tools to assess what is working in their local communities.

PIP supported by the 4-R process is adaptable to completing action research, Flashlight, CBA, SPARC, MEASURE, and even RAMP. The point is that the process is designed to promote the learning power and relational wellness of the engaged professional.

Reflective Moment 9.5

Phase 4: Community Assessment and Reflection

Step 7. Actions are assessed and results discussed with the learning community.

PIP Activity: Using the 4-R process or PIP, please describe your change steps and address the following questions: What are your results? Who are you sharing the results with? Graduate students, helping professionals working in your school, administrators, parents, students, the school board, or other key community members? What is the format? How is the format conducive to improving student support?

Celebrating the Living Story

Completing an action research project, a Flashlight, SPARC, MEASURE, or RAMP is an important part of celebrating what has been accomplished in moving toward addressing some challenge or reaching some goal related to building a school community that fosters learning power and relational wellness. Still, after completing the project, sharing the results, it is necessary to view the process as ongoing. Work in the schools is the work of life; it must continually be watered, nourished, and weeded if it is going to continue to grow. Documents cannot be pointed to as, "this is it." Perhaps, that was "it" when doing what was done at a particular point in time. Now, it is a matter of documenting what is happening in the moment and where the effort is to move the students toward greater learning power and relational wellness. This does not mean that old practices are tossed away because new lessons, interventions, and programs are necessary for the sake of newness; it means that what is done has to be kept alive and vital to the needs of the students, the school, and the community being served. Thus, the process always returns to the positive core in lifescaping: what gives life to what is done, for all the stakeholders in the school and community. By publishing your lifescaping efforts, you celebrate the steps taken toward improving the learning power and well-being of your students. If you are interested in publishing or want to share how your lifescaping efforts were shared, let us know at lifescapingproject@gmail.com. The Lifescaping Project is working with the Taos Institute to develop platforms that provide a voice to those professionals using appreciative inquiry and action research to give life to schools, communities, and organizations.

Reflective Moment 9.6

Phase 4: Community Assessment and Reflection

Step 7. Actions are assessed and results discussed with the learning community. Actions are reflected upon and efforts are shared with the larger community, e.g., with all students in the school, department members, school community, school board, college or university class, etc. Results may also be used as part of a document that highlights action and practices of helping professionals in the schools, such as Flashlight PowerPoint, SPARC (Support Personnel Accountability Report Card), etc. Feedback from stakeholders and interested parties is reflected on and used, if possible.

PIP Activity: How are you going to celebrate what you have accomplished or learned? How has the students' learning power or relational wellness been enhanced by your collaborative actions?

Continuous Improvement and Inquiry

Continuous improvement concentrates on building upon the best traditions within the organization and by focusing on enhancing the positive core in the school's lifescape. How does this build upon our best traditions? There are obligations to oneself as an individual, one's school, and to the community where that school is located. The 4-R process is about remaining alive ecologically as an engaged professional within schools as systems, beginning by building relational connection, dreaming about possibilities in relational dialogues, taking relational actions, and moving into relational action and reflection. Like life, the process is one we are challenged to enter into fully and with passion, celebrating our successes and learning from our most glorious failures, always wondering, "What other, more beautiful pathways could we build or create to make this a better place?"

Reflective Moment 9.7

Phase 4: Community Assessment and Reflection

Step 8. The strategy is adapted accordingly via learning community reflection. What would you/we do differently?

Step 9. Action is taken to put the revised strategy into practice, and necessary steps are repeated. A time frame is set to revisit what has been done and the strategy being implemented. Like expiration dates on milk cartons, a time is set in order to revisit, reassess, revise, and renew practice.

PIP Activity: Write one to two pages about what you would recommend to improve what you have done and steps you or others should take in the future. This writing can be done individually, in small groups, or with the learning community that participated in the collaborative action. Whatever format(s) is chosen, there should be a venue for collaborative sharing and revision of the strategy(s).

Reflective Moment 9.8

Continuous Improvement or Never-Ending Story

- How does this build upon our best traditions?
- What can we celebrate?
- What other, more beautiful pathways could we build or create to make this a better place in this never-ending story?

Advocacy and Participatory Leadership

Participatory leaders are cheerleaders and innovators during PIP Phase 4: Community Assessment and Reflection and AI Phase 4: Relational Assessment and Reflection. In order to initiate Phase 4 of the PIP or AI, participatory leaders are advised to reflect on the four skill-sets described in the wellness domain: performative focus, vital engagement, self-reflectiveness, and relational connectedness. Performative focus calls for personal and social competence in sharing new forms of life within the community of practice and with the larger community. Vital engagement calls for being excited about what has been learned and about the prospect of addressing even one small problem by offering a new form of life. Self-reflectiveness opens advocates to bricolage and makeshift adjustments that will be necessary to move the work forward into new ways that inform the new forms of life and the never-ending learning story that define schools. Finally, relational connectedness calls upon leaders to be thankful to the relationships formed and even challenged during the entire project.

In this chapter, participatory leaders are most concerned with the results of a project in a never-ending story directed toward making the school where the project is implemented a more vibrant learning community that fosters learning power and promotes student well-being.

Chapter Summary

This chapter concentrates on assessment: AI Phase 4: Relational Assessment and Reflection and PIP Phase 4: Community Assessment and Reflection. Actions are assessed in order to determine what worked and what did not work, and hopefully, to find what worked best given the intervention. In other words, AI Phase 4: Relational Assessment and Reflection and PIP Phase 4: Community Assessment and Reflection are about learning, not about harsh judgment. What was learned? What were the results of a project that is concerned with making one thing better at the school where it is implemented? Where do we go from here? What do we build upon?

Part III

Lifescaping in Action

Told in Participatory Inquiry Process (PIP) and AI 4-R Phases by Student Advocates Working in Schools

Introduction

Part III is about applications. Part III provides four examples of how the participatory inquiry process (PIP) and appreciative inquiry (AI) process were implemented within specific school communities. It is important to note that each of the chapters was written at different points when the PIP and AI approaches shared in this text were being developed. We recognize the limits of not focusing on our current "best practices," but we also wanted to capture how the lifescaping projects shared in this book capture a dynamic process concerned with creating new forms of life in specific schools. The authors of these chapters did not have the benefit of having this entire book in the format that you find. As editors, we have maintained a stance that the beginning professional's voice matters and we have tried to make sure not to edit or shape the individual author's thinking; we wanted readers to see how lifescaping new forms of life in schools is eco-relational. We have asked the authors to align their chapters with the current PIP and AI phases as much as is possible.

First, in Chapter 10 Molly Griffin shares her participatory inquiry from the perspective of a professional-in-training in a school counselor graduate program. Second, in Chapter 11 Lisa Maibaum shares how she used appreciative inquiry as a director of special education tasked with a district mandate to address disproportionality. Third, in Chapter 12 Katie Messina, a counselor and instructor, shares how she works with first generation students transitioning from high school to community college using the tools of AI as well as PIP. Fourth, in Chapter 13 Lisa Davies is a site administrator who builds upon the culture; she shares how she uses a dialogical approach to engage teachers as co-researchers in participatory action research based on an issue identified through a participatory inquiry process; her discovery of the overlap with appreciative inquiry came after reflecting upon her own process and professional development. We share her work to illustrate how conversations about PIP and AI can evolve and inform lifescaping efforts in schools.

10 A Write Way Intervention

Successful Transitions into the Ninth Grade

Molly Griffin

Phase 1: Initiating Conversations and Identifying Challenges

Step 1

In the fall of 2010 as a second year school counselor-in-training I began my fieldwork at Hillview High School in Hillview, California. I began my work with my fellow school counselor-in-training, Gizelle Roberson, by shadowing our supervisors, credentialed school counselors Joe Kinney and Dorothy Dunlap. At the start of each school year, high school counselors begin by conducting senior check-in meetings with twelfth grade seniors to assess each students' academic progress thus far, advise on classes needed to meet graduation requirements, college entry requirements, and ways to remediate courses. Often times during senior check-ins, we would hear twelfth grade seniors say, "I didn't realize those classes I took my freshman year really mattered!" After hearing this statement, we discussed with Mr. Kinney and Ms. Dunlap the idea of us counselors-in-training acting as freshman support counselors. Our supervisors felt that there was a need for freshman support counselors; we were assigned this informal title and got to work.

Step 2

After seeing the need for guidance for staying on track for high school graduation, we began discussing the different interventions we could implement at Hillview High School to best share this information with students. With our emphasis on freshmen, we discussed ideas such as quarterly "check-ins" with all students who had one or more F grades in a class. The check-ins would be designed to assist students in setting goals for any classes students were failing and discuss the importance of earning credits and passing their high school classes. However, in doing so we realized that we would not be reaching all students and providing all students with such valuable information about their high school careers and beyond. We realized that the information needed to be prepared and delivered to all freshman students so that there would be an equitable system in providing high school graduation and college preparation information to all students.

Professor and school counseling supervisor, Dr. Rolla Lewis, approached us with the idea of implementing a guidance curriculum for all ninth grade students that would provide each student with the information and skill building opportunities to foster understanding of the requirements for graduation, the calculation of high school credits, and the development of problem solving, decision making, and goal setting skills. Dr. Lewis had drafted and implemented a guidance curriculum called "A write way" (1999), which is a transitional guidance curriculum focusing on high school graduation readiness and requirements, college readiness information, and high school transition skills. The guidance curriculum also fosters resiliency, assists and encourages students to create a powerful learning story about themselves, and assists with the transition into high school. Dr. Lewis shared the curriculum with us, and, with his blessing, encouraged us to use whatever pieces of the curriculum we felt would best support our initiative to provide graduation readiness and high school skills to the freshmen students at Hillview High School.

Phase 2: Engaged Inquiry

Step 3

Dr. Lewis shared with us how "A write way" (1999) had been used in the past to provide high school students with the opportunity to use structured narrative assignments to assist them in developing their own individualized story of school, identify success and areas of weakness, and uncover the skills of goal setting, problem solving, and decision making. We felt that this curriculum, with minor tweaks, would be a great starting point for implementing the type of program we were looking for. We strongly felt that there needed to be a career component to the curriculum, as well as a college preparatory piece to assist students in comprehending that the classes they begin as a freshman are not only required for high school graduation but also are college preparatory classes and are required by four-year universities for admission.

Step 4

As we began to map out the components of our curriculum, Dr. Lewis also encouraged us to view the implementation of "A write way" (1999) as an opportunity to collect data throughout the school year and track students' progress, willingness to participate, and their understanding and acquiring of skills. Dr. Lewis continued that there could also be a possibility of assessing the impact of a transitional guidance curriculum over time using longitudinal data. With this encouragement, we simultaneously began to research, plan out our desired comprehensive curriculum, and evaluate the data tools we would use to measure the dissemination of information. We felt it was important not only to assess students' understanding of information, but also students' support systems, how they set goals and how they viewed and planned for success.

As we began researching the trends in school-wide data, using information from the School Accountability Report Card (SARC, 2009), we found that in the 2008–2009 school year, 83 percent of seniors graduated from Hillview High School. Thus, 17 percent of the 2009 senior class was not eligible for high school graduation and post-graduation opportunities. We then reviewed the quarterly progress report grades of all freshman students and found that over half of the 436 freshman students were receiving D or F grades at the first progress report marking period. While reasons may vary as to why 17 percent of the 2009 seniors were not eligible for high school graduation, we realized that there seemed to be a missing link in the dissemination of information to freshman students about the importance of their ninth grade classes and the requirements for high school graduation and four-year college entrance requirements. Both Gizelle and I felt that it was important for all students to have the opportunity to understand and plan for not only high school graduation but also for post-secondary educational opportunities. Often times twelfth grade students' options can be limited on post-secondary educational opportunities due to the lack of planning in the earlier high school years. We felt that the sharing of information had to be equitable; every student has a right to know and plan for the post-high school future.

As researchers, we developed our own assessment tool to capture data in these areas (see Appendix K: Assessment Instrument: A Write Way Curriculum Questionnaire). Additionally, we felt very strongly that students should have the opportunity to evaluate the curriculum and us as their counselors delivering the curriculum. We designed a comprehensive curriculum assessment tool similar to the Outcome Rating Scale (ORS) and Session Rating Scale (SRS) tools developed by Miller and Duncan (2000). Using additional resources and conducting literature reviews, we began to incorporate additional information and techniques to be used throughout implementation. We both felt strongly that there needed to be an action or activity piece to each lesson while finishing the activity with the structured narrative writing assignment.

Additionally, we both are proponents of *Reaching all by creating tribes learning communities* (Gibbs, 2006) and felt that it would be important to provide students with the opportunity to discuss community agreements and to make sure these agreements were very clearly explained and agreed upon by all students. At the beginning of the first lesson, the four community agreements outlined by *Tribes learning communities* (Gibbs, 2006) of active listening, no put downs, respect for yourself and others, and advocate for your own learning were explained to all students by giving definitions and examples. We also felt that it was important to place the students in groups (or tribes) for group work and activities. As school counselors-in-training, we explained that the groups that the students had been placed in were like small tribes, and that the students, teachers, and counselors were a collective community and that community agreements for our tribes and community had to be established. In *Tribes learning communities*, author Jeanne Gibbs states that defining community agreements "is important for the students in your classroom to enter into a discussion of what they need in order to feel safe, or trusting, in a group" (Gibbs, 2006, p. 85). The students responded well to the community agreements and were receptive when encouraged to hold each of their tribe members accountable if they broke one of the agreements.

Phase 3: Collaborative Action

Step 5

As we began to observe the senior check-ins and hear students say how much they wished they knew about high school before they started high school, we began to realize that this was our purpose as freshman support counselors. In working with Dr. Lewis and his suggestion and encouragement to use "A write way" (1999), we felt that this could be and would be the type of tool that would help inform and transition freshman students into high school and allow them additional successes. Our hope was that as they got to their senior year, counselors would not be hearing, "I wish I knew how important that ninth grade class was!" Our hope was to give them the tools to begin to reflect on their current academic practices with the hopes that they would begin to see their future more clearly and thus begin lifescaping their own future.

As we began planning, researching, and developing "A write way" (1999), we worked closely with Dr. Lewis to discuss and evaluate each lesson of the curriculum. This process happened over time; we met with our advisor almost weekly to discuss additional options for lessons, research, and ways to collect data. Dr. Lewis encouraged us, as two researchers, to discuss the protocol of data collection at Hillview High School, the use of consent forms, and the possibility of some day writing about our findings.

As we began to adopt and adapt "A write way" (1999), we decided on eight lessons to implement and would be implementing each lesson once a month (see Appendix K). We felt that with the knowledge from these eight lessons, the freshman class (class of 2014) would see greater graduation rates than the previous years' classes and have a greater understanding and preparedness of high school graduation requirements and post-secondary college entry requirements.

Step 6

"A write way" (1999) guidance curriculum was first proposed to our supervising guidance counselors at Hillview High School. After establishing that there was a need for this type of guidance curriculum, we reached out to the four freshmen Health/College Success In Progress (CSI) teachers to ask for their participation in allowing us as school counselors-in-training to come into the classroom once a month to implement monthly lesson plans. The health classes were suggested because every freshmen student was required to take the Health/CSI class. The Health/CSI teachers along with the principal and counseling staff were pleased to support the implementation and evaluation of the curriculum. We arranged a schedule so that we would implement eight lessons over the course of the school year to all 436 ninth grade students.

Phase 4: Community Assessment and Reflection

Step 7

1. *Data Collection*: We used a variety of assessment tools for the curriculum, but one of the most powerful is the Write Way Curriculum Questionnaire (see Appendix K: Assessment Instrument). It consists of four questions: 1) in high-school my goal is to; 2) what do you want to do after high-school?; 3) I have achieved ____ goal(s) I have set for myself; and 4) someone who can help me achieve my goal is. As researchers, we used this tool at the beginning, the middle and the end of the curriculum.

2. *Data Analysis*: In addition to reviewing the data collected by our research tool which helped us to gather both qualitative and quantitative data at the beginning, middle and end of the curriculum, we also read through every structured narrative for every student after each lesson. We felt that if we were going to ask students to open up to us about their successes and struggles academically and personally, we had an obligation to read what they had to share. This allowed us to not only see how our students viewed their future, the number of goals they achieved, etc., but also how they viewed themselves and their life story thus far. It was a wonderful way to connect with our students and hear their individual voices.

Additionally, we both felt that it was important to share this information with not only their counseling team at Hillview High School, but with the Health/CSI teachers, and administrators. We completed an action plan, comprehensive lesson plan, and results report with all research and data and shared them with each stakeholder at Hillview High School.

3. *Results*: The majority of students indicated that in high school, their goal is to "achieve excellence." We hoped that the curriculum would

cultivate a learning environment where all students would feel that they could aspire to and achieve greater goals for themselves in high school and beyond. We incorporated this data when we wrote the Support Personnel Accountability Report Card (SPARC) for the 2010–2011 school year at Hillview High School. A copy of the award winning SPARC and the certificate of completion was also mailed to the superintendent of Hillview Unified School District.

4. *Limitations*: Having taken a research methods class, we were aware of the limitations of our guidance curriculum if we wanted to collect data from the student population. Dr. Lewis assisted with the process of completing the Internal Review Board (IRB) paperwork to be approved by California State University, East Bay as researchers in our graduate program. The IRB did not agree that passive consent forms would be appropriate for the approval of data collection at Hillview High School. Instead, we were required to obtain written consent from every student and their parent or guardian that the students' responses and surveys could be used for research and publication. After rewriting the consent forms and submitting all research tools, "A write way" (1999) guidance curriculum and data collection tools were approved by the IRB. With the approval from the principal at Hillview High School, we worked with the Health/CSI teachers to distribute and collect all of the consent forms. Consent forms were also translated into Spanish, as 40 percent of the Hillview High School population was Spanish speaking. As soon as the consent forms were signed, we began administering surveys and questionnaires to collect data.

5. *Reflection*: Throughout the year, we began to share our findings with our site supervisors. We read through every student's structured narrative writing after every lesson; students shared some very powerful and personal stories that often led to further discussion with that student alone. In our weekly discussions with Dr. Lewis, we were also able to share in the success and struggles of implementing the curriculum. As the students began to get to know us as their counselors, they were more open to sharing personal struggles and successes in their structured narrative writings. This allowed the students to reflect upon themselves, the successes they had had, the mistakes that they had made, and how to set goals for the future. Thus, they were beginning to conduct their own personal lifescaping. We came to see that even though these ninth graders were only just beginning their high school career, most were craving the opportunity to learn and plan for their future. Gizelle and I often reflected that we really enjoyed being in the classroom with the students every month. We could see that not only were we providing a foundation to lifescape for our students and the school, but we were lifescaping in our work as counselors-in-training. The progress our students began to make truly changed and informed our counseling practice.

With the encouragement of Dr. Lewis and our site supervisors, we presented our findings to all Hillview Unified School District counselors at a district-wide counselors meeting in May, 2011. We were invited to present our findings in the research methods class as part of the Educational Psychology department at California State University, East Bay. Additionally, we also presented our research at the SOLES Action Research conference in San Diego, CA in May, 2011.

This action research project strongly assisted in the development of our professional practice by challenging the researchers to have a participatory role in the development and implementation of a component of a school counseling program. The implementation of "A write way" (1999) transitional guidance curriculum helped us build competency in collaborating with teachers, administration, counselors, and other school staff to put into practice a curriculum that addresses a specific area of need for all students. Additionally, the development of a transitional guidance curriculum and the results allowed us to see the effects of our work. Through these conversations with students, parents, teachers, and administrators, we began the work of lifescaping; the work of adapting our perspective that emerged through the participation in implementing a transitional guidance curriculum.

Lastly and perhaps most importantly, viewing the data from the curriculum can be used effectively to support the development of a comprehensive school counseling program, by showing how important it is to dedicate some time to the social/emotional aspect of the students' experiences because it directly correlates with their academic success. Hillview High School can use the data to show the community and all other stakeholders what different types of preventative measures are being taken by the school to decrease high school dropout rates.

Step 8

If we were to implement "A write way" (1999) again, there are a couple of things that we would do differently. We wished we would have met with the specific teachers before beginning the curriculum to go over some of the needs of the resource students in their classes, so as to be able to accommodate their specific disabilities more effectively. As researchers, we also would have added an additional evaluation to each lesson to be able to evaluate each session instead of the curriculum as a whole. Lastly, we would have had the students complete all questionnaires and evaluations in the computer lab so that all of the results were automatically generated, instead of tallying the results by hand.

In the final months of the school year, we began to consider how "A write way" (1999) would and could be implemented in years to come. With a strong focus on building a system-wide freshman transition initiative, Hillview High School could see a vast difference in graduation and college going rates. With the help of Dr. Lewis, we reached out to soon to be second year school counselors-in-training who would be placed in high school settings for their fieldwork experience. We encouraged two trainees to join them for "A write way" (1999) lessons in the classrooms to see the implementation in action. They also discussed the research, the evaluation tools, and the specifics of the curriculum in hopes that the two future trainees could successfully implement "A write way" (1999) guidance curriculum.

Step 9

It has been over a year since those initial conversations and we do believe that pieces of "A write way" (1999) guidance curriculum were used to support the new ninth grade students. Gizelle is now a counselor with Hillview Unified School District and often stops by Hillview High School for meetings with counselors, and often times she will see some of the freshman students she worked with; they still recognize her and remember her and Molly as "their" freshman counselors. It is great to know that our presence has impacted students' lives and hopefully their educational journeys.

Longitudinal data of those students who participated in "A write way" (1999) show a significant greater number of students from the group being retained in their sophomore and junior years than that of the class ahead of them (see Appendix K). In the 2011–2012 school year, the class of participating students' percentage of being retained was 94 percent compared to the 88 percent of the class ahead of them. In the 2012–2013 school year, the class of participating students' percentage of being retained was 90 percent compared to the 80 percent of the class ahead of them.

Additionally, in the 2012–2013 school year, approximately 79 percent of the participating class was on track for high school graduation compared to all other Hillview High School students, where 74 percent were on track for high school graduation.

11 Advocating with Appreciative Inquiry (AI)

Lisa Maibaum

Phase 1: Relational Connection

In March of 2010, Highland High School District (HHSD) was identified by the California Department of Education (CDE) as having Significant Disproportionality (SD). African-American students accounted for approximately 3.5 percent of the total district population; however, this demographic made up 11 percent of the total special education population. Although this system-wide issue was identified for the district by an outside government agency, a simultaneous process of data evaluation was previously conducted at the high schools. The required corrective action proposed by the California Department of Education launched HHSD into examining their issues with disproportionality, not just in the special education arena. System-level initiatives are typically not received well when mandated by an outside agency. Therefore, in order to help the staff make sense of the CDE citation itself, it was critical that HHSD administration present the internal district data that was reviewed by CDE. The decision to focus on issues related to disproportionality, specifically the over-representation of African-American students in special education, was framed to staff as not only a mandate from CDE that required action, but a moral imperative.

I was selected by the special education director to lead Highland High (the most diverse school in HHSD; thus, the most affected) in understanding issues related to disproportionality. In addition to gathering, analyzing, and presenting data for the staff, providing direct pre-referral intervention for students was also expected. Finally, as a school psychologist, and thus serving as a "gatekeeper" to special education, I had to carefully watch all special education referrals of African-American students throughout the district. These were the only guidelines provided to me, which made the role extremely daunting. I was pleased with the level of vagueness, however, because it allowed my mind to explore all possibilities, and dream of an ideal way to provide service delivery in the general education environment. I was also pleased that, in the efforts to quickly eliminate our disproportionality issue, I was not told to simply start re-assessing and exiting African-American students who were already benefitting from Individual Education Plans (IEPs). Such a directive would have presented both ethical and moral dilemmas and confounded the already daunting task.

In addition to the lack of blueprint I was given for this endeavor, the fact that I was alone on this project posed another major challenge. How was I going to raise awareness at the high school about our district's challenges with disproportionality? How was I going to redefine my role for the staff and build relationships with general education teachers? Would I have the support of the administration? To start, I decided to approach the site administration at Highland High about joining the weekly teacher–leader meetings as a way to build relationships and begin conversations related to this work. Adding equity and challenging disproportionality in this school required a lifescape that fostered genuine dialogue. These meetings were already the venue in which data collection had begun taking place which was revealing a major achievement gap between our African-American students and students of other ethnicities. Grade distributions by course and ethnicity had already revealed that our African-American students were under-represented in Advanced Placement courses, over-represented in the lowest level Algebra classes, and were the group most likely to fail that Algebra class. These teacher–leader meetings were also the venue in which items such as the master schedule were discussed and rally planning was conducted. Although there were many meetings with agenda items that were not related to disproportionality, I attended every single meeting; simply to maintain my presence and role within the group, maintain my relationships, and keep our issues of significant disproportionality salient on everyone's mind. Lifescaping this intense and controversial issue requires patience and elegance; maintaining my physical presence in the group was symbolic of my persistence and commitment. Over time, the teacher–leader meetings began to be the venue to organize and plan staff development days. To my benefit, this group also led planning of staff development days. By spring, the group moved to define an expectation that staff have at least one workshop, "chalk-talk" or panel presentation related to issues of cultural diversity and disproportionality.

Phase 2: Relational Dialogue

After identifying the appropriate venue and key allies to discuss issues regarding disproportionality, the next step was to frame the conversation using research-based findings related to issues of race and achievement in schools. As I began researching, I first looked to my professional organization, the National Association of School Psychologists (NASP), for data related to race, achievement, and disproportionality. References from NASP led me to a plethora of relevant articles that I ultimately arranged into a PowerPoint presentation for staff. Finally, supported by my school district administrators, I attended local presentations and workshops related to these issues.

First, I wanted to highlight for the staff the direct correlation that supportive relationships and school connectedness have with achievement. A caring teacher–student relationship is positively and significantly associated with a higher GPA across ethnicities (Crosnoe, Johnson, & Elder Jr., 2004). However, there is a "support gap," in that Euro-American and Asian-American students often report receiving more teacher support than their African-American or Latino peers (Jia et al., 2009). Furthermore, research suggests that there are racial disparities in school connectedness. African-American students report lower levels of connectedness to teachers than other ethnicity groups (Karcher & Sass, 2010). African-American students also report the lowest levels of school connectedness compared with all other ethnicity groups (Jennings & Tran, 2009).

The concept of cultural mismatch was the second point to highlight to staff. School culture is often based on mainstream European-American culture which can disadvantage students from diverse backgrounds (Sullivan, 2010). Children whose household culture does not match the school culture face a disadvantage upon entering a school that is maintained by "taken for granted" practices and cultural norms that are not explicitly instructed to disadvantaged students (Sullivan, 2010). Cultural mismatch can be seen in curriculum as well. There exists a lack of curriculum in which African-American students can find the intellectual achievements of people who look like themselves represented (Delpit, 1995). The notion of cultural mismatch applies to behavior as well; especially as it applies to the *emotional disturbance* criteria for special education. The problem of disproportionality in special education, specifically the over-identification of racially diverse students as emotionally disturbed, may be the result of widespread and chronic failure to value cultural differences (Sullivan, 2010).

In terms of behavior, it is important to remember that *different* does not mean *disabled*. Cultures differ in what constitutes appropriate behavior. In school settings, behaviors that deviate from the cultural norm tend to be pathologized and result in special education referrals. Some deviations in behavior represent differences in values and learned behaviors, rather than some kind of disability or dysfunction. In fact, many behaviors that are deemed "inappropriate" may be adaptive in home contexts. Impassioned and emotive reactions can be interpreted as combative and argumentative (Townsend, 2000). Vavrus and Cole (2002) analyzed videotaped interactions among students and teachers, and found that many referrals were less the result of serious disruption than what the authors described as "violations of . . . unspoken and unwritten rules of linguistic conduct" (p. 91), and that students singled out in this way were students of color. African-American and Latino families are more likely than their

European-American peers to receive expulsion or out of school suspension as consequences for the same or similar problem behavior (Skiba, Horner, Chung, Rausch, May, & Tobin, 2011). If there is a mismatch between students' behaviors and the norms or values of the school, efforts to "fix" the problem can lead to special education referral (Sullivan, 2010).

The goal in presenting this data to the staff at Highland High was to provide some background regarding issues of equity and achievement. Also, the hope was that teachers would reflect on their own practices in the classroom, and how those practices and assumptions impact ethnically diverse students who are academically struggling. Ultimately, I was striving for all teachers to engage in personal reflection regarding the learning lifescape of their classrooms.

After providing this theoretical framework to the staff, it seemed clear that the next step was to analyze our school-wide data. The question driving this data was the following: Do racial disparities in special education mirror similar disparities in rates of discipline, achievement, and placement in AP classes? In 2008 African-American students accounted for 3.3 percent of district population yet accounted for 27 percent of district suspensions. In regards to the California High School Exit Exam (CAHSEE), 95 percent of the total population passed on the English Language Arts (ELA) section on their first attempt; however, only 66 percent of African-American students passed on their first attempt. Similarly, regarding the CAHSEE Math section, 93 percent of the total population passed on first attempt; however, only 66 percent of African-American students passed on first attempt. Finally, data revealed under-representation of African-American students in Advanced Placement courses. Twenty eight percent of the total population was enrolled in at least one Advanced Placement class, while only 7 percent of the African-American population was enrolled in at least one Advanced Placement class.

This data demonstrated to the staff that racial disparities at Highland High were not unique to special education. Communicating this data to staff was necessary in order to convey the reality of disproportionality as it applies to the entire school system. Otherwise, disproportionality concerns may have been interpreted as a problem for only the special education department to address.

Phase 3: Relational Action

After reviewing and sharing the school-specific data, I needed to engage with the staff and students regarding how to address the problem. Of course I had my own ideas and plans forming with regards to intervention. I knew it would not be received well if I simply imposed my intervention plan without listening and inquiring as to what the staff and students thought would be effective. Lifescaping is collaborative; it is not about enforcing an agenda. I continued to meet weekly with the teacher–leader group, share data with teachers at staff development days, and review special education files of our African-American students to make sure non-discriminatory assessment procedures were being followed. Finally, the chair of the Math department (who turned out to be one of my biggest allies) arranged for a panel discussion of African-American students to take place at one of our staff development days. All staff were required to rotate through the panel discussion. Target questions for the students covered school climate and experiences in the classroom. Finally, a survey was conducted asking all struggling students (identified by their enrollment in an academic support class) what makes them feel comfortable versus uncomfortable in the classroom, and what helps them to succeed in the classroom. The data from this survey was compiled, the results were shared at the teacher–leader meeting, and then disseminated to all staff.

Phase 4: Relational Assessment and Reflection

After data review, it was clear that racial disparities were a school-wide issue, permeating most aspects of the school. This led me to the conclusion that simply providing more "gatekeeping" of African-American students into special education was not going to be a satisfactory intervention. Monitoring referrals to special education was going to be part of the job, but certainly not the primary role. After consulting with the special education director, we agreed that we needed to target African-American students who were at risk of entering special education. We figured that if we could intervene early (as soon as they enter ninth grade), and provide tailored intervention based on specific need, those students would have a better chance of succeeding both academically and behaviorally in the general education environment.

We agreed to partner with the feeder schools to gather data regarding incoming African-American students (without IEPs) who were at risk of struggling both academically and behaviorally. I decided to attend the ninth grade summer transition program (which was a support already put in place for incoming ninth graders who were at risk) to build relationships with students, observe behavior, and review classwork samples, to gain a sense of what kind of support they would need upon entry in the fall. After a caseload was identified, students began receiving intervention immediately after school started. The variety of supports offered were: individual counseling, group counseling, ninth grade transition groups focusing on behavioral needs, and literacy groups (doing guided reading and writing activities using CAHSEE prep material). I provided the above interventions as well as case management and ongoing consultation to the students' teachers. The case management was, in effect, an effort to mirror the kind of support offered in special education. I also followed the students for two years and faded support during their junior year.

Results from the first intervention year revealed a reduction in initial
assessments of African-American students. Twenty percent of all initial assessments were African-American students (down from 56 percent). Suspensions
among African-American students were also down; only one suspension was
for defiance/disruption, which was the targeted discipline code (due to its
subjective nature). During the intervention year, African-American students
accounted for 12 percent of the district suspensions. This was down from
27 percent the previous year. These results were first shared with the special
education director, then the teacher–leader group, and finally, disseminated
to the staff. These results proved that progress was being made; thus, it led
to the decision to continue the program in its current format. These results
also highlighted that our district was able to make progress related to over-
representation *without* simply exiting incoming African-American students
from special education.

The development of the disproportionality program and its initial results
were shared with the superintendent and the school board by the special
education director. It was critical for the superintendent and the members
of the school board to hear the progress made by this program. The stakeholders needed to understand the important progress made on such a
substantial undertaking such as addressing disproportionality. The hope
was also that the district would continue to fund this program by
maintaining the school psychologist position. At present, this position and
intervention program still exists, even though we have satisfied our mandate
and are no longer deemed "significantly disproportionate" by state standards. Equity and disproportionality issues are now an added dimension to
the lifescape of Highland High.

After learning of my unique role in addressing over-representation of
ethnic minorities in special education, I was approached by my professor
from graduate school, Dr. Greg Jennings, to come and speak to the second-
year school psychologist cohort at CSU, East Bay. The purpose was
twofold. He wanted me to share how data was used in approaching a large,
system-wide issue. Also, he wanted me to share information regarding
over-representation of ethnically diverse students in special education, to
bring their awareness to the issue. Next month will be my second visit
to my alma mater to present on this topic.

My professor, Dr. Jennings, also approached me about collaborating
on a presentation for the National Association of School Psychologists
(NASP) conference in San Francisco in February 2011. The topic of over-
representation and significant disproportionality was addressed through
the context of how to foster culturally relevant school climates. Finally,
my special education director approached me about presenting with her
at the Association of California School Administrators (ACSA) in Mon-
terey, CA in January 2012. This presentation specifically addressed issues
of equity and how Highland High responded to the state's citation of being
"significantly disproportionate." At both NASP and ACSA, almost all our

audience members admitted that their districts were struggling to address issues of over-representation of ethnically diverse students in special education.

Looking back on how the disproportionality program was implemented, I would make a few changes in how the information was disseminated to teachers and other school staff. Conversations and relationships were built solidly at the district level, and even at the site administrative level; however, I wish I had more time to talk with teachers. This program directly impacted them; as I was asking these teachers to consult with me (a non-teacher!) regarding how to provide more support to targeted students. A few teachers took this program offensively, as if the district was telling them they were not doing enough for their African-American students. Enhancing my relationships with the teachers (not just the teacher–leaders, who were only one person representing an entire department) would be the main area on which I would focus. I would like to conduct focus groups with the teachers, or engage in fishbowl discussions, and do teambuilding activities to build relationship and awareness to issues of equity. The relational component is so critical and cannot be emphasized enough when undergoing systemic reform. Another area for improvement is the method of the consultation that took place. Many times, due to busy schedules, consultation was taking place through email, where intentions can be misunderstood. Committing to making in-person appointments or phone consultations is something to prioritize moving forward.

The disproportionality program still exists at Highland High, in a fairly similar form. Although run by another school psychologist, it is still thriving, and achieving similar success on a variety of outcomes. The new school psychologist heeded my advice about building relationships with teachers and being mindful of delivering consultation in any other manner rather than in-person or via phone. She has strengthened our relationships with the feeder schools, and we have more information regarding our "at risk" incoming ninth graders. The biggest change in the program is that the school psychologist is focusing on academic and behavioral interventions, and allowing the school-wide counseling program (comprised mostly of MFTs and psychologist interns) to provide the individual and group counseling to address emotional needs. Currently, Highland HSD is starting to navigate and introduce Response to Intervention as a district-wide initiative. The disproportionality program is being looked to as a guide in this process, as it is a model for how to provide tailored intervention to students in the general education environment.

12 High School to Community College Transition Group

Katie Messina

Introduction

As a counselor and instructor, I have worked in the San Francisco Bay Area at the high school and community college levels for over ten years; in my work at both levels, I have had the opportunity to witness, first-hand, the struggles that many of my students continue to face. The transition from high school to community college can be challenging for many students. Many high school students arrive at community college without clear direction, major/transfer plans, or knowledge and familiarity with the community college/transfer process. The result is that many of them drop out and fail to attain a certificate, Associate's Degree, or transfer to a four-year university. My observations of my current and former students in addition to the research I have conducted regarding transfer and graduation rates at California community colleges clearly illustrate this troubling trend.

This action research project was conducted during the 2013–2014 academic school year while I was a second-year graduate student at California State University, East Bay. I am not using the actual name of the high school where the project was conducted; for the purposes of this study, the high school will be referred to as East Bay High School (EBHS) and the local community college will be referred to as San Francisco Bay College (SFBC). The names of all individuals have also been changed. EBHS is a small public charter high school of approximately 500 students; most students are low-income and first-generation college-going. While the school reflects the surrounding district schools' demographics and incoming student achievement rates, the small school size and strong college-going school culture, combined with high levels of support, have led to high academic achievement rates by graduation. During the previous academic school year, EBHS had a 96 percent graduation rate for students finishing in June, and a 99 percent graduation rate by August; 97 percent of students attended a two- or four-year college in June after graduation. Every year approximately one-third of the graduating senior class attends a local community college, and the vast majority of students choose SFBC, the local college. SFBC is a medium sized public two-year community college that serves approximately 14,000 students from the surrounding areas. Like EBHS, SFBC has a very diverse student body and many students are low-income and are the first in their families to attend college.

I believed the best way I could work within the context of my high school was to improve the counseling services for our community college-bound seniors. Using the lifescaping construct and the participatory inquiry process (PIP), the goal of my research study was to better provide all community college-bound students at EBHS with a clear path to SFBC, as well as the necessary background information and knowledge to be more successful students once they transitioned to community college.

Lifescaping and the Participatory Inquiry Process

Lifescaping is the engaged action to bring about greater learning power and/or well-being in the school community. In this project, I endeavored to lifescape my school and district to offer a more supportive environment for community college-bound students to flourish. The main lifescaping tool utilized in this action research study was the participatory inquiry process (PIP), a theoretical model designed to guide practitioners in generating knowledge and conducting practical research within the school contexts in which they work (Lewis & Winkelman, 2014). The PIP was used as a framework to identify challenges, pose solutions, identify resources, build a collaborative solution, and evaluate results within a high school context.

Literature Review

Studies show that graduation and transfer rates are lowest at community colleges that have the highest percentages of low-income, first-generation students. In contrast, community colleges that have more affluent, higher performing students tend to have the highest graduation and transfer rates (Gandara, Alvarado, Driscoll, & Orfield, 2012). Examination of local California Bay Area community colleges illustrates this point clearly. The following data were collected from the College Measures website, and show the combined graduation and transfer rates within three years. It should be noted that many students do graduate and/or transfer in longer than three years, and data collected within a seven-year time span show slightly higher rates. Community colleges located in more affluent areas with high performing feeder high schools showed graduation/transfer rates of 68–72 percent. In contrast, SFBC has only a 38 percent graduation/transfer rate. Other surrounding community colleges that also have high concentrations of low-income, minority students showed graduation/transfer rates around 30 percent (CollegeMeasures.org).

Because I work at schools with high percentages of students who are low-income and first-generation college-going, I wanted to look specifically at what factors influenced community college transfer and graduation rates within this demographic. My research led me to an excellent and relevant study conducted by UCLA's Civil Rights Project that examined factors at the high school and community college levels that influenced transfer rates among California's under-represented students (Gandara et al., 2012).

According to the UCLA Civil Rights Project study, influential factors at the community college level included a strong transfer culture, special programs, efforts to reduce remediation, access to knowledgeable counselors, and connections to local colleges. Special programs such as Puente, Adelante, EOPS, Umoja, MESA, and TRIO are all designed to help students who are low-income, first-generation, or from under-represented groups transfer to four-year universities. Research shows that students enrolled in these programs transfer at about twice the rate of other students. However, special programs tend to serve a small percentage of students at the community college, and the study recommended looking into ways of expanding such programs to reach more students.

The need for remediation is also a huge factor for many community college students coming from low-performing high schools. Successful community colleges created summer bridge programs, Freshmen Year Experience programs, and other creative "refresher" classes or workshops to help reduce the need for remedial courses. The role of counselors was specifically emphasized; the study mentioned that schools which had a philosophy that "all counselors are transfer counselors" tended to be more successful than programs with just one or two transfer counselors. A welcoming and supportive environment for students of color, especially with counseling, was also cited as an important factor. On a programmatic level, the availability of transferable courses and connections/pipelines to local four-year colleges were also cited as important (Gandara et al., 2012).

At the high school level, important factors cited included outreach counseling from local community colleges, a stronger emphasis on basic math and English skills, stronger high school counseling support, and field trips or orientations at local community colleges. The study showed that much of what the only community college counseling high school students received was from outreach counselors from local colleges. Many community colleges send counselor representatives to feeder high schools to present on financial aid, the matriculation process, and the transfer process. They often also included outreach ambassadors, who were current community college students, to talk about their experiences. The study also mentioned that field trips and orientations at local community colleges helped students feel connected and informed. This study, in addition to many others, cited the need for strong academic preparation at the high school level. The better prepared in English and math students are, the fewer remedial classes they will have to take in college, and the more quickly they will be able to graduate and transfer (Gandara et al., 2012).

Community

This action research study was conducted over the course of the 2013–2014 academic year at EBHS with a group of twenty-eight high school seniors, almost one-third of that year's senior class. The lead school counselor and I used school data to identify the target group. For this study, we decided to focus solely on all seniors who were either not four-year university eligible or who were borderline four-year eligible based on the CSU eligibility index which combines GPA and SAT/ACT scores. Although there were other additional students who were four-year eligible, but were considering community college instead, we decided we would provide support to them in alternate ways.

The Participatory Inquiry Process (PIP)

Phase 1: Initiating Conversations and Identifying Challenges

The first phase of the PIP process focuses on examining the school environment and available data, and then initiating conversations with key stakeholders to identify challenges or areas of need (Lewis & Winkelman, 2014). My research was conducted at EBHS, a small public charter high school of approximately 500 students, where I had previously worked as a teacher and was working as a school counselor intern when this study was conducted. Because it was my seventh year working at the school, I was already quite familiar with the school community and its programs. The school had developed a strong comprehensive school counseling program under the leadership of the head counselor, Dr. Reyes. There was a strong focus on preparation for a four-year college; however, in the past there had been less support for community college-bound students. Because of this, Dr. Reyes stated that one of her goals for that year was to increase the level of support for our community college-bound students. When I mentioned my interest in working with that group, she immediately agreed and said she would be happy to have me take the lead on that project.

I was particularly interested in working with this group of students because I was also working as a counselor intern at the local community college, SFBC. At the time, I was working with the Puente Project, part of the special programs division of counseling. The Puente Project was originally designed to increase the transfer rates of Latino/a students from community college to four-year universities. Currently, the Puente Project is based on three main components: counseling, English and writing development through coursework focused on the Latino/a experience, and mentorship and community leadership. The Puente Project works closely with a cohort of students to build strong relationships and support to help them develop the skills they will need to succeed in community college and transfer to a four-year university. Generally, Puente students transfer at twice the rate of other students (Puente Project, 2014). I believe this is because of the strong counseling and mentorship components of the program. It also has a strong cultural component and helps students build a sense of community on campus, as well as develop close relationships with faculty from similar backgrounds to their own.

Because I was working at both the high school and community college levels at the time, I was uniquely equipped to closely understand the needs of students as they made the transition from high school to community college. Part of my interest in this project also came from the conversations I had with students at both levels. At the high school level, some of the community college-bound students voiced concerns about not getting as much help as they needed from counselors, feeling confused and unsure about what they wanted to do, and being unclear about the transfer process. At the community college level, many students reported still feeling "lost," even after two or three years there. Many of these students said they were still unsure of their major and/or transfer plans and were just taking classes without having a clear academic or career plan. I also observed that the students who seemed to be most on-track towards graduation and/or transfer were those enrolled in special programs like Puente, EOPS, or MESA.

After thinking about these student comments and observations, I started wondering about what "lifescaping" we could do at the high school level to help better prepare students for success at the community college level. The lead counselor and I brainstormed some ideas and thought about how we could continue to build on the systems we already had in place. So, she and I worked with the rest of the counseling team to begin developing the framework for a high school to community college transition group. I discussed the idea with the principal and he was also very supportive and gave us the "go-ahead." Our main goal with the group was to help students successfully navigate the SFBC matriculation process, familiarize them with the transfer process and the resources available at community college, and help as many students as possible enroll in special transfer programs.

Phase 2: Engaged Inquiry

Phase 2 of the PIP process focuses on gathering data and research to identify what resources already exist, what is working, and what changes need to be made within the school context (Lewis & Winkelman, 2014). I began by researching and reviewing the literature to see what factors help students make the bridge between high school and community college. I found there was a lot of research on factors that helped students succeed at community college and transfer to four-year colleges, but I found little research on what high schools could do to better prepare students. Then I found a study conducted by UCLA's Civil Rights Project that examined several California high schools and community colleges that had high levels of success graduating and transferring low-income minority students (Gandara et al., 2012). This study significantly informed my project because it specifically addressed the same student population that I work with and cited ways to best meet their unique needs. In reflection of the Multicultural Counseling Competencies, I wanted to make sure our project specifically met the needs of our students (see Appendix L for specific standards addressed). Many of the elements at the high school level were things that we could do at my site for our students. I discussed my ideas with Dr. Reyes, the lead counselor, and together we identified the students and developed the workshop components.

We used school data to identify the target group. For this study, we decided to focus solely on all seniors who were either not four-year university eligible or who were borderline eligible. We decided to focus on this group because we felt they needed the most support and we could design targeted group interventions to best meet their needs. We identified a group of twenty-eight students in total, which was almost one-third of that year's senior class. Through our individual conversations with these students we identified that twenty-three planned to attend SFBC, the local community college, and five planned to attend another area community college. We decided we would have the SFBC-bound students complete their matriculation process, which lays out an easy set of steps to follow and grants them priority registration status. We had students complete this process the prior year as well, so we already had some supports in place to build upon. We decided to start with what we already had and expand our services where we could. We agreed that we would conduct pre- and post-program surveys and collect key outcome data to assess the effectiveness of our program.

Phase 3: Collaborative Action

Phase 3 of the PIP process focuses on creating an intervention and taking actions to put the agreed upon strategy into practice (Lewis & Winkelman, 2014). Dr. Reyes and I established that the main goal was for all community college-bound seniors to complete *all* matriculation steps, apply for special programs, and begin community college with resources, knowledge, and a plan. My secondary goal was also to help address the stigma many students felt was associated with community college. I wanted our students to feel like attending a community college was a viable and good alternative for them. Guided by the ACA Advocacy Standards, I wanted students to feel empowered and to show them how to advocate for their own education once at community college (see Appendix L for specific standards addressed).

Together, Dr. Reyes and I developed the framework for a series of eight workshops that would cover community college and transfer basics, career/major exploration, the matriculation process, financial aid, and special programs (see Appendix L for outline of each session). I wanted to make sure the workshops also included opportunities for presenters to talk about their experiences of being successful at a community college. Together, we outlined what the workshops should include, and then I put together the workshop presentations and materials and led them with students.

Phase 4: Community Assessment and Reflection

The fourth and final phase of the PIP process focuses on gathering data and evaluating the results of the project. The results are then discussed and recommendations and adjustments are made accordingly (Lewis & Winkelman, 2014). In order to gather the necessary data, I designed several tools to assess the effectiveness of our High School to Community College Transition Program. I designed a survey to give to all the students to assess their educational goals, understanding of community college, and transfer steps, as well as levels of counselor support during the process. We also created a spreadsheet to track outcome data such as matriculation steps completed, special program applications, and assessment results.

I completed the University Institutional Review Board (IRB) Protocol, and once we had board approval, we began the workshops right away. We completed all eight workshops with students, including individual and small group follow-up meetings as needed. I conducted the workshops after school and during the school advisory periods so that students did not have to miss any academic class time. We conducted pre- and post-program surveys and gathered all of the outcome data for all the students who participated in the study. Survey and outcome data showed the following program highlights:

- By the end of the program, 100 percent of students had established an educational goal (i.e., obtain an Associate's Degree or transfer to a four-year university), compared with 63 percent on the pre-program survey, and 92 percent of students had selected "Transfer to a 4-year university" as their primary educational goal, compared with 48 percent on the pre-program survey. Additionally, 95 percent of students had selected a major of interest by the end of the program.
- 100 percent of SFBC-bound seniors completed the matriculation program components on time including: online college application, financial aid application, Math and English assessments, orientation, group counseling session, and class registration.
- On the assessments, the following percentage of students placed at college level or one semester below college level: Math—61 percent, English—83 percent.
- On a scale of 1–5 (1 = not supported, 5 = very supported), the average score was a 4.3 in terms of how well supported students felt by counselors during the community college application process.

- 87 percent of all students applied for at least one special program at SFBC (i.e., Puente, EOPS, etc.)

The data collected show a number of important results from the High School to Community College Transition Program. First, by the end of the program, all students had identified an educational goal and the number of students planning to transfer to a four-year university increased to 92 percent. Similarly, 95 percent of students had identified a major of interest. This is significant because it shows the High School to Community College Transition Program helped students establish a clear educational goal and major that will improve their chances of working towards that goal once they reach community college. Second, all SFBC-bound seniors completed all matriculation steps and registered for classes by the end of May. Third, the assessment results indicate that a majority of students were placed at or one semester below college level in English and Math, which will greatly increase their chances of completing community college course requirements in a timely manner. However, increasing the number of students who assess directly into college level Math and English is still an area for future growth. Fourth, students reported feeling a high level of support from their counselors as a result of the High School to Community College Transition Program. While feelings of stigma associated with community college were more challenging to assess, students made comments indicating they felt support from counselors and administrators in their decision to attend a community college. Lastly, the majority of students applied for special programs that will help them get extra counseling support and help them stay on track with the transfer process.

At the end of the school year, we evaluated the program's effectiveness based on the data we gathered. I revised the program based on our discussion and made everything easily adaptable for other counselors to use. The counseling team has continued to use and improve the program we created and they have shared our work with the other schools in the charter network as an example of how to support community college-bound seniors. As a counseling team, we felt very excited about the program and the ways in which we were able to lifescape our school and district in order to offer improvements in support for our community college-bound seniors.

Conclusion

The High School to Community College Transition Program is an example of how a high school counseling team was able to use the lifescaping construct with the participatory inquiry process as a framework to effectively identify an area of student need and then propose, implement, assess, and revise a practical student support program. This research study also shows the need for more comprehensive support systems in high schools and community colleges to help students successfully navigate this challenging and crucial transition.

13 Algebra as a Civil Right

Increasing Achievement Through Participatory Action Research and Appreciative Inquiry

Lisa Davies

Robert Moses states, "Mathematics Education is a civil rights issue" (2001, p. 5). Moses argues that children who are not quantitatively literate may be doomed to second-class economic status in our increasingly technological society. Unequal numbers of poor, African-American, and Latino students drop out of mathematics and perform below standard on tests of mathematical competency, and are thus denied both essential skills and a particularly important pathway to economic and other opportunities. This chapter describes the role of participatory action research in developing the understandings and practices of Algebra teachers determined to improve the achievement of African-American male students. An appreciative inquiry approach served as the foundation for the collaborative process. The principal modeled qualities of relational connection as she engaged teachers and students as co-researchers in the inquiry.

Future Forming Purpose

This participatory action study evolved from the desire of Algebra teachers and their principal to better serve underperforming students, particularly African-American males, in an urban middle school. For the purpose of improving student achievement, four teachers volunteered to serve as co-researchers: completing surveys, being videotaped, contributing in lesson debriefings, and sharing their experiences in final interviews with their co-researcher principal. As the collaborative inquiry progressed the following questions emerged: What practices promote academic success for African-American males in Algebra? How do teachers define, promote, and recognize student engagement (particularly among African-American males) in Algebra lessons? Does collaborative inquiry impact teacher attitude, belief, and teaching practices to increase the success of African-American males in Algebra?

The Intersection of Theoretical Frameworks and Participatory Action Research

This study was grounded in Adult Learning Theory. Just as schools should be designed as learning communities and around the principles of how children learn, so should teacher development be structured around how adults learn (Hunt, 2003). Jackson (2009) describes adult learning theory as humanist, cognitive, and constructivist. This perspective and theoretical framework is intricately connected with the methodology. Action research was purposefully selected as a democratic and critical, constructivist approach to the study (Herr & Anderson, 2005).

Participatory Action Research Design and Methodology

This study utilized a participatory action research design to capture teachers' experiences with collaborative inquiry in the area of Algebra instruction. Classroom visits were videotaped by the principal co-researcher using an iPad, then shown to the co-researchers in debrief sessions. During the debrief sessions the teacher co-researcher who was videotaped shared the content of the lesson and explained the teaching strategy used. Co-researchers offered comments and feedback to the teacher about the lesson and teaching. The principal co-researcher interviewed each teacher co-researcher after the final debrief session. During the interviews, the co-researchers discussed their participation in the study, shared their learning and interpretation of student engagement, and generated questions to be used with the student focus group. An Algebra student focus group was convened from students enrolled in the observation classrooms. The students were randomly chosen by the co-researcher principal to answer questions about their experiences in their math class.

Discussion of the Participatory Action Research and Appreciative Inquiry

This inquiry illustrates an ongoing cycle of the 4-R AI process as teachers along with their principal engage in relational dialogues, relational actions, relational assessment and reflection. The student voice is captured in focus group conversations that further support the professional learning and action to improve instructional practice.

Table 13.1 captures the sample responses from and to the four teachers (identified as Young, Hart, Garza, and Smith) who de-privatized their practice and engaged in critical discourse on their pedagogy and use of instructional strategies.

The following sections briefly describe outcomes of this inquiry process including: the development of constructivist leadership; the promotion of productive collaboration; the identification of effective teaching strategies; and a shared definition of student engagement.

Table 13.1 Teacher and Student Responses

	Young	Hart	Garza	Smith
Debrief on videotaped lessons *self* feedback	That lesson is like the best lesson I have all year, I got the materials and I've got the thinking I use choral response but didn't get enough engagement	I talk too fast It is hard to understand me	Some will say, oh, it's childish in terms of age appropriate strategies I want to provide access for them	The process itself caused me to reflect more on my own instruction/ practice, learning from the others. I should be doing this better
Debrief on videotaped lessons *peer* feedback	(You) used the visuals, the juice, and technology Pair share Try it, if we are nervous we sabotage the trial of the strategy, try it with different classes . . . a totally unique experience	(You) used the technology, visuals and maps This was definitely solid lesson, solid for sure, better than when I was teaching it. What I did was mediocre compared to your lesson. Wait time	(You) used tapping and repletion of exponent power as re-engagement tool not as a method to teach exponents. They (students) are not ready for just memorizing new rules; they're ready for let's practice and see what this looks like	(You) used drumming and rhyme to help students' memorize steps. Pair share Too long on one problem, hard to follow the math
Teacher interview responses *self* reflection (**Post-lesson debrief cycle**)	Insightful for myself I gained (knowledge) about their teaching practice and my teaching practice, what they thought was informative, what they thought was not informative	It gave me different ideas for changing up my own lessons and how other people are getting students engaged It gave me a lot of different ideas and techniques for teaching different concepts	It gave me (the opportunity) to share ideas with my colleagues, get their opinion on what I am doing	Visual aids caused me personally to think of the problems differently, deepened my understanding and my understanding of students

Table 13.1 continued

	Young	Hart	Garza	Smith
Student focus group comments regarding each teacher's instructional practices	"Mr. Young already has it down right now" "Have the other teachers watch Mr. Young"	"She is new, she is like an elementary teacher so she is not used to teaching, this is why Mr. Young is giving her instructions on how to deal with the kids" "She goes too fast over the Algebra, she goes over more stuff, when I ask questions, she tells me we are running out of time, by the end of the period, I forget my questions"	"Kids keep asking what, how do you do that?" "When the answer is right there, pacing gets slower, and I start to drift off" ". . . he slows down too much"	"Kind of fun some days, we do partner work some days, we make Algebra posters, like we look in our textbooks, copy it down, then he puts it on the wall, if you don't know something you can look at the posters, we use drumming and rhyming to review for tests"

Developing Constructivist Leadership

"Constructivist leadership," both learning and leading (Lambert, 2003) was evident in this study. Together the participants were able to construct meaning through inquiry, participation, and reflective dialogue. The participants generated the collaborative inquiry of the study. The co-researchers led the dialogue and learned from each other's teaching as they built the inquiry base to inform their teaching and student learning. The development of these teacher–leaders will build capacity for the collaborative inquiry to continue to grow in this school. Teachers from other departments at this middle school are already asking whether their team can use the model of collaborative inquiry used in this study.

Promoting Productive Collaboration

In this participatory research study the conversations moved away from traditionally blaming the students and their parents for lack of achievement to coherently analyzing instructional practices, sharing different perspectives, and creating a safe space where everyone's feedback was appreciated and valued.

Identifying Effective Teaching Strategies

In their lesson debrief sessions, teacher co-researchers determined that the use of interactive strategies—including think pair share, hands-on work with manipulatives, visuals, technology, and productive group work—were effective. They found that Algebra content could be made relevant to students' lives through lessons such as problem posing based on a trip to Los Angeles and the use of real liquids to illustrate a connection to mixture problems. They observed that the strategic use of rhythm, rap, and rhyme, tied to curricular objectives, captured students' attention and increased students' active participation in the classroom.

Defining Student Engagement

In their final interviews all four teacher participants defined student engagement as "getting students to think." They described the importance of Algebra instruction that moves beyond simply solving equations to higher order activities. For instance, instead of proclaiming "this is the solution," one co-researcher proposes asking the students, "is this the solution, why or why not?"

Significance of the Inquiry

> "She goes too fast over the Algebra, she goes over more stuff, when I ask questions, she tells me we are running out of time, by the end of the period, I forget my questions." (African-American male Algebra student)

One of the most significant findings in this inquiry was the clear alignment between the descriptions of teachers' practices provided by the student focus group and the co-researcher teachers' reflections during debrief and interview sessions. The teacher of this student identified her tendency to "talk too fast," but more importantly the co-researcher collective continually addressed the use of relevant instructional strategies to develop students' conceptual understandings and enable teachers to stop "racing through" content. This inquiry allowed co-researcher teachers as well as the co-researcher principal to see the classroom through "different eyes"—the students' eyes (Cahill, 2007).

This inquiry was a successful conduit in creating an environment of learning, a professional learning community. Through this process participants built trust within their Algebra teacher community. The teachers were eager to learn from each other and were willing to de-privatize their practice by being videotaped and participating in collaborative inquiry around student learning. Their willingness to maintain their rich collaborative inquiry culture morphed into regular classroom observations of each other. The participants began using their preparation periods and lesson planning to infuse culturally responsive teaching strategies to engage African-American students. Learning is not only a means to an end; it is the end product (Wenger, 2006), which was the final product for the participants as they took a collective responsibility for learning and changing.

For Further Inquiry

Even though the study focused on African-American males, the student assessment data were analyzed on African-American males, and each of the videos included a focus on African-American male students, race was not discussed. The conversations during the debrief sessions addressed "all students" and did not focus on African-American male students. Though the videos captured African-American male students who were clearly off task and not focused at times, there was no direct conversation about any of these students in the debrief sessions. Without direct prompts and focus on the African-American male students, the co-researchers, including the African-American principal, reverted to speaking about their students as a whole without disaggregating the African-American males as the focus. This pronouncement confirms that race continues to be a challenging topic for discussion.

This chapter is not the final statement on the impact of participatory action research and appreciative inquiry as a vehicle for increasing achievement in Algebra of African-American males, but it does provide a promising starting point. Several insights and recommendations are offered in this study, but our "thirst for knowledge remains unquenched." We will continue to study how to best serve African-American males until the achievement gap is closed.

14 Conclusion
Bringing AI and PIP Together

... the research scientist looks forward not only with equanimity but also with excited interest to the fundamental changes which later research will bring.

(George Herbert Mead, 1932, p. 41)

Creative emergence occurs along the margin of neither/nor: neither too much nor too little order, neither too much nor too little disorder.

(Mark C. Taylor, 1993)

A conclusion assumes some closure. Yet, given the radical openness of the universe, there are always gaps where things have not been said, new interpretations are possible, and something new or new forms of life open up how "things are." We end up living in never-ending stories directed toward lifescaping and future forming the world that we want. That is the strength of both appreciative inquiry and the participatory inquiry process. Each project never ends; each engagement ends with a new vantage point and, hopefully, offers new forms of life that enhance the eco-relational space where they have been enacted. Each school-based project is a continuous, never-ending process that concentrates on life-enhancing practices directed toward fostering student learning power and relational wellness in the entire school and community. Completed AI and PIP projects exist as markers and measures but the intention is to enhance development and foster new forms of life as a lifelong process that calls for learning power, which is about cultivating specific knowledge, skills, and attitudes, and relational wellness. Actions guiding AI and PIP projects are oriented toward connecting with the people and the local life-systems where we live and work in this flow of life.

Advocacy, Action and Reflection Revisited

The chapters in Part III illustrate lifescaping and future forming in action. Each chapter provides us with the opportunity to revisit the advocacy stance proposed in Chapter 1 from a new vantage point. We see, we hear, we are not quiet about what we see and hear. We learn with and from our graduate students who embody, and thus further define, the role of student advocate. Together we bring about new forms of life by enacting via the lifescaping processes inherent in action research and appreciative inquiry.

As student advocates we choose to see. To see is to understand, realize, grasp, recognize, observe, perceive, comprehend, and consider. We can look closely or we can look away. Molly Griffin chose to recognize that 17 percent of high school seniors did not meet the high school graduation requirements. As she further examined the data, she found that more than 50 percent of freshmen students were receiving D or F grades on their first progress reports. Lisa Maibaum observed that while African-American students comprised 3.5 percent of the district population, 11 percent of the special education student population was African-American and, in 2008, 28 percent of students suspended were African-American. Katie Messina considered the 38 percent graduation rate in the community college where she served, in contrast with the 68–72 percent graduation rate of the community colleges serving students from more affluent communities in the surrounding area. Lisa Davies realized and pointed out that while teachers initially identified the low performance of their African-American males in Algebra as the focus of their inquiry, these teachers chose to discuss "all students" in their lesson debrief conversations. In each inquiry the student advocate continued to look into, not away from, the challenges presented.

To hear is to catch, get to know, perceive, receive, gather, make out, and pick up. As student advocates we not only choose to hear, we create opportunities to listen deeply, like anthropologists listening to learn. Molly used "The write way" structured narratives to hear the voices of individual students. Lisa Maibaum coordinated a panel discussion with African-American students and conducted a survey of what makes students feel comfortable and uncomfortable in the classroom. Katie conversed with individual students to identify their matriculation needs. Lisa Davies co-facilitated a focus group of students who clearly articulated their Algebra teachers' strengths and areas for growth and professional development. The students' analysis correlated with teachers' lesson debrief conversations. In each inquiry the student voice was shared with teachers and others who could then engage in lifescaping dialogues.

In this work, we are not quiet about what we see and hear. Student advocates take action based on what we see and hear. We proceed, labor, perform, and often replace traditional practice with innovations and new forms of life in the educational settings where we find ourselves. How we do what we do matters. We do not act alone; we form relationships and collaborate. Molly worked with the principal, Health/College Success teachers and counseling staff, all of whom supported piloting the "write way" curriculum with 436 ninth grade students. Lisa attended the ninth grade summer transition program to build relationships with students and learn more about the support programs already in place. Katie brainstormed with the lead counselor and the counseling team to develop the framework for a High School to Community College Transition Group, based on conversations with high school and community college students. As principal, Lisa Davies videotaped lessons and scheduled time for teachers to meet, yet teachers took the lead in analyzing lessons, learning from one another how to improve their service to students. The appreciative inquiry and the participatory inquiry process keep us honest; there is always further action to be taken or refined in our school communities.

In the introduction we stated that this book is not for armchair reading. We offer concluding remarks but, as student advocates, you will write the next chapters. What issues do you see that are not being addressed in your school community? How will you use the tools provided to "unearth" the stories that are not currently being heard? How will you take collaborative action to create conditions that will better serve students? We invite you to share your work with us as you walk this path.

In conclusions we look for pithy summaries. Perhaps we can offer Five Maxims for lifescaping and future forming practice:

First, we exist in biological and social ecological systems. We are connected to each other and all of life. It is vital to respond with wisdom and mindfulness within the biological and social systems we are part of, and not separate from as we flow through life. AI and PIP are designed to foster greater compassion, participatory, and democratic action within school systems as learning communities.

Second, we exist in developmental, relational contexts, and narratives. Be careful about riding a high horse. We are all students in life and the ultimate story is about how we contribute to enhancing and enriching the lives of those around us as compassionately as possible.

Third, we exist in a world filled with possibilities, endless conversations, dialogues, and decisions. Listen, value the multiple and diverse voices around us, take baby steps, persevere, and be curious and in awe of the possibilities inherent in life. AI and PIP are designed to keep the conversation going and the narrative(s) of the school continually evolving in a compassionate direction.

Fourth, we can choose artistic, action-oriented solar ethic in our embrace of life. Do not be a lump. This life is everything we are experiencing. Engage life as creatively as possible and take action toward celebrating and enhancing this gift with others. The current social drift toward self-absorbed hedonistic and materialistic abandon is contrary to a social ethic; the solar ethic is a radical call for a compassionate response to injustice, greed, and the destruction of human and biological ecosystems that we are all part of, as well as a path that calls helping professionals to create the conditions for others to live up to their potential. Create new forms of life with others. AI and PIP embrace fully engaging the organizations where we work in ways that help as many people as possible to live up to their potential as learners, workers, and citizens.

Fifth, recognizing our limitations and challenges, we can calmly choose to have our professional practice informed and guided by a sense of responsibility and ethical engagement. We have a responsibility to engage others in dialogue and ethical engagement rather than in arguments that alienate and entrench. A small win and a baby step in the right direction might be enough in the moment. AI and PIP are about calmly engaging school communities in responsible, compassionate, and ethical action directed toward helping all students learn to live, to learn, to work, and to contribute to a democratic society.

Like Voltaire at the end of his classic *Candide* written in 1789, this book will end by saying, "we must cultivate our gardens" (Voltaire, 1956, p. 189). Yet it is important to note that the "American" garden was different from the French garden, and becoming more so as the United States defined itself as a nation. Our founding fathers were obsessed with gardening and used garden metaphors to inform their political actions. They also found personal peace and comfort in designing their gardens to fit their unique ecosystems and landscape (Wulf, 2011). The many different gardens and gardeners of the new nation brought about diverse ways to cultivate and also new plants to bring to market. The land and the people were connected.

We must engage in dialogues and action collectively in our local settings in order to make our lifescape more vibrant, alive, and productive. That is the work at hand and the challenge in every school and community attempting to promote the learning power and wellness of all youth, and for that matter, all citizens. That is what it means to be a citizen of the United States because this nation is an experiment in democracy. In the United States, we live an aspirational ethic. Since Thomas Jefferson wrote "All men [sic] are created equal" the aspirational ethic guiding the best of its citizens in the United States expanded the notion of equality to include ex-slaves, women, gays, and every new ethic group coming to our nation. We do not forget that Thomas Jefferson was a slaveholder, and a very flawed person, but in terms of the founding fathers, we can recognize and appreciate George Washington was the single founding father who mandated that his slaves be freed upon his death in 1799. We do not have to deny the brutality and history, but we can appreciate that justice and compassion take place one act at a time.

But like every nation, community, school, or living organism, life is an evolutionary process that never ends as long as it exists. We must continually cultivate the gardens of democracy (Liu & Hanauer, 2011) and compassion in our communities (Gilbert, 2009). Our collective participatory practice can cultivate our families, schools, and communities in ways that produce the most energetic brothers, sisters, learners, and citizens, because more than anything else, a vibrant democracy depends upon the positive relationships, compassion, knowledge, skills, and aptitudes of its people.

Humans will live and die regardless of human theories. Still, this was a text about theory and practice. Critically, however, some theories developed by humans are better than other theories, and every approach to action necessitates "epistemic humility" about what is known and requires individuals to convey tentativeness in a world where possibilities are the best people can go on (Taleb, 2007, p. 190). Whatever our human constructions, the world moves on with or without humanity's chatter. Part of our epistemic humility must embrace the notion of ecosphere, a term illustrating the interdependence of all living beings (Bender, 2003, p. 20). Ultimately, as bumper sticker wisdom implores, nature bats last. We are part of, not apart from, this world. We are part of interlocking life systems that include air, water, earth, and animals; our common ecosystems are our life-community to which we all belong (Bowers, 1997, 2003; Capra, 2002; Goleman et al., 2012; Leopold, 1949; Spretnak, 2011; Williams & Brown, 2012). Humans are part of and citizens of social and biological systems and ecologies; individual selves are not separated, regardless of any myths or personal existential fears. In fact, Naess (1988, 2002) asserts that self-realization is tied to seeing oneself as part of the larger social and biological ecology where people exist as living beings in dialogue with each other and connected to the world they are part of.

The eco-relational approach is a way of viewing human beings as embedded in chronological, social, and biological systems where they develop in time, as social beings, and as part of the natural world as members of life-communities that include plants and animals. Still, each person is born at a unique historic moment and contextual place characterized by distinctive cultural connections within any variety of bio-logical and social ecologies. By integrating theory, research, and best practice, the eco-relational approach to building learning communities in schools is geared toward assisting helping professionals improve their practice, conversations, and actions over time by developing their current strengths, school and community assets, and their students' desire for authentic engagement in their own learning and in their own relationships, both personal and professional. The eco-relational approach views people as participating in and related to interlocking social systems, or social ecologies (Bronfenbrenner, 1979; Conyne & Cook, 2004; Lewis, 2011; Goleman et al., 2012; Prilleltensky & Prilleltensky, 2006; Skolimowski, 1994; Sterling, 2001; Williams & Brown, 2012). Understanding social and ecological connectedness is crucial; people are part of, not separate from, the life-systems they are embedded in and surrounded by. Humans participate as members of a living planet and human life-communities (Bowers, 1997, 2000; Capra, 1996, 2002; Goleman et al., 2012; Leopold, 1949; Skolimowski, 1994; Spretnak, 2011; Sterling, 2001; Williams & Brown, 2012).

There is not a singular story. There are story ecosystems. There is never one story. Every story has infinite alternative stories. Thus there are vast networks of stories told and stories that are possible in the story ecosystems where humans find themselves. The aliveness of and gaps in language cannot be over-emphasized, nor can the understanding that all stories have gaps, different possibilities for interpretation, and openings for new or alternative understandings (Boyd, 2009; Briscoe et al., 2009; Bruner, 2002; Gergen, 2009; Goleman et al., 2012; Lakoff & Johnson, 1999; Mehl-Madrona, 2010; Monk et al., 1997; Peavy, 2004).

The eco-relational approach is dialogical and understands the self as constantly in flux, constantly changing depending upon the dialogues and relationships the person is engaged in during their life. In other words, individual meaning moves; meaning is never fixed; it is relational, evolving, and subject to critical reflection. As such, meaning is always contestable, and different, alternative meanings are possible (Gergen, 2009; Linell, 2009; Peavy, 2004).

This text has offered a perspective and tools for developing stories in schools that promote the notion of schools as learning communities concerned with fostering well-being and learning power as a way of life.

In this text we have presented lifescaping as a form of action directed toward cultivating learning power and well-being in schools, organizations, and communities. Both lifescaping and future forming move research away from being a descriptive summary or an attempt that supposedly mirrors reality toward action research as an engaged creative and continuous process directed toward making schools, organizations, and communities more beautiful places for living and learning. The strengths-based eco-relational change practices to be implemented in school communities shared in this text offer tools for creating schools as beautiful places for promoting well-being and learning power.

We have also asserted play that flows and liberates us from ways of being that oppress or hold us back to "the way things are." Lifescaping is not a sad-faced, grind-it-out endeavor. Lifescaping actions using PIP and AI can be viewed as play activities where we free ourselves to become the producers, builders, and creators of our lives in the moment; where we find flow as we learn to become producers, builders, and creators of learning communities that cultivate well-being and learning power by playfully engaging in PIP and AI lifescaping and future forming actions in collaboration with others.

We wish you the best in constructing a better world for all. With this text, you have tools to make your school, community, and organization a better place. This book offers the tools to help you engage in a continuous developmental process where you are obligated to tap your courage to look, listen, speak, and engage in dialogues designed to lead to actions intended to help student learning power and well-being. But any action is never perfect; all actions must be assessed for efficacy, reflected on, and improved in ways that enhance professional practice, student engagement and learning, and human relationships as living and dynamic processes. We never fully arrive at some endpoint or closure; we are living and learning beings. Let us know about your lifescaping efforts; contact us at lifescapingproject@gmail.com.

Websites

Action Research in School Counseling: www.schoolcounselor-advocate.com/
Action Research International: www.scu.edu.au/schools/gcmar/ari/arihome.html
Action Research Network of the Americas: www.arnaconnect.org/working-groups/working-groups-interest/school-counseling
Appreciative Inquiry: http://appreciativeinquiry.cwru.edu/intro/conference.cfm
ARexpeditions: http://arexpeditions.montana.edu/docs/about.html
ASCD Whole Child Initiative: www.ascd.org/whole-child.aspx
Building Learning Power (BLP): www.buildinglearningpower.co.uk/
California Safe and Supportive Schools: http://californias3.wested.org/
Caring School Community: www.devstu.org/caring-school-community-implementation-resources-documents
Center for Ecoliteracy: www.ecoliteracy.org/
CESCal Flashlight Builder: www.cescal.org/flashlight.cfm
Collaborative Action Research Network (CARN): www.esri.mmu.ac.uk/carnnew/
The Cloud Institute for Sustainability Education: www.sustainabilityed.org
Collaborative for Academic, Social, and Emotional Learning (CASEL): www.casel.org/home/index.php
Compassionate Mind Foundation: www.compassionatemind.co.uk
Edible Schoolyard: www.edibleschoolyard.org/
Education for Sustainable Development Toolkit: www.esdtoolkit.org/
Educator Competencies for Personalized, Learner-Centered Teaching: www.jff.org/publications/educator-competencies-personalized-learner-centered-teaching
EZAnalyze: www.ezanalyze.com
Flashlight Builder: www.cescal.org/flashlight.cfm
Greater Good Center: http://greatergood.berkeley.edu/
Highlander Research and Education Center: www.highlandercenter.org
Institute for Community Research: www.incommunityresearch.org/about/about.htm

International Resilience Project: www.resilienceproject.org
Living Values Education: www.livingvalues.net/index.html
MindsetKits: www.mindsetkit.org/
The Ontario Action Researcher: www.nipissingu.ca/oar
Performing the World: www.performingtheworld.org/
Public Conversations Project: www.publicconversations.org
Resilience: Building a World of Resilient Communities: www.resilience.org/
Restorative Justice Constorium: www.restorativejustice.org.uk/
Restorative Justice 4 Schools: http://restorativejustice4schools.co.uk
School Reform Initiative (SRI): www.schoolreforminitiative.org/
Self-Compassion: www.self-compassion.org
Social Publishers Foundation: www.socialpublishersfoundation.org/
Sunnyside Environmental School: www.pps.k12.or.us/schools-c/profiles/
    ?id=191
Support Personnel Accountability Report Card (SPARC) at: www.
    calcareercenter.org/sparc
Taos Institute: http://taoslearning.ning.com/
Taos WorldShare Books: www.taosinstitute.net/worldshare-books
UCLA School Mental Health Project: http://smhp.psych.ucla.edu/
University of San Diego Action Research Center: www.sandiego.edu/soles/
    centers-and-research/action-research/index.php
WestEd: www.wested.org/cs/chks/print/docs/hks_resilience.html
Youth Participatory Action Research and School Counseling Practice:
    http://files.eric.ed.gov/fulltext/EJ1034747.pdf

Appendix A
Professional Competencies and Ethics

COUNSELOR ADVOCACY COMPETENCIES:
http://counseling.org/resources/

COUNSELOR MULTICULTURAL COMPETENCIES:
http://counseling.org/resources/

ETHICAL STANDARDS FOR SCHOOL COUNSELORS (American
School Counselor Association)
http://schoolcounselor.org/asca/media/asca/Ethics/EthicalStandards2016.
pdf

SCHOOL PSYCHOLOGY PRINCIPLES FOR PROFESSIONAL ETHICS
(National Association of School Psychologists)
www.nasponline.org/standards/professionalcond.pdf

Appendix B
An Ecological Model (School Counselors)

Table B.1 An Ecological Model (School Counselors)

Ecological Level	Program Development Examples
Ecosphere Life systems, bioregions, etc.	• Understanding world as living system; projects related to understanding global warming, etc. • Recognizing that ecological disasters cause demographic shifts; relief efforts for disaster area, i.e. New Orleans, Haiti, etc.
Ethnosphere Diverse cultures; language, values, national boundaries, gender roles, etc.	• Understanding diverse human cultures throughout the world, making new immigrants welcome at school. • Understanding how students who are fleeing from conflict may require special culturally sensitive programs and additional support.
Macrosystem National identity, international agreements, socio-economic status (SES), national wealth, national resources, war, etc.	• Identify community, culture, gender roles, media, peers, etc. influences on current program and practices. • Understanding how international agreements, cooperation impact students' lives, especially new immigrants. • Understanding and helping students impacted by parents, family, relatives, and friends serving in the armed forces.
Exosystem Public Policy	• Identify ecological influences of education and school policies on counseling program, counselors' role, etc. • Review school counseling licensing and credentialing rules, state policies, and state rules and laws related to school counseling. • Facilitate stakeholders working together to define comprehensive school counseling program within district. • State funding for edible garden projects.

continued

Table B.1 continued

Ecological Level	Program Development Examples
Mesosystem Relationships among microsystems	• Facilitate school counseling program's connections with community resources and other schools with programs via asset mapping. • Include parents, families, teachers, administrators, and community members in school counseling program advisory. • Identify and consider mesosystemic relationships and influences. • Network of edible garden projects in region.
Microsystem Family, friends, school, church, team, work	• Facilitate students' awareness and identification of ecological factors impacting school success. • Facilitate students in identifying one adult mentor or success coach. • Develop edible garden project at school.
Individual Gender, cognitive factors, biological factors	• Facilitate students' awareness of learn to live, learn to learn, learn to work, and learn to contribute. • Facilitate students' ability to define school success and set goals to achieve it. • Facilitate students' abilities to identify personal strengths and attributes related to school success. • Learning about cooperation, biology, and cooking by participating in edible garden project at school.

Source: Lewis (2010). Used with permission.

Appendix C
Promoting Vital Engagement and Eco-Relational Change

Table C.1 Promoting Vital Engagement, Relational Wellness, and Learning Power

Appreciative Inquiry (4-R) and PIP Phases	PIP Change Steps 1–9	Relational Focus	Inquiry and Guiding Questions	Core Counseling Skills
Relational Connection (4-R) Initiating Conversations and Identifying Challenges (PIP)	Systems Change Steps 1, 2, (9)	Connecting to individuals, school, and community. Define positive core. Defining core value. Dialogue with others. Listening to current and past stories.	What are the school's strengths? • What can we do to promote wellness, academic, personal/social, and career success for all students? • How can I embody "vital engagement?"* • Who are we, collectively and professionally? • What are we doing to promote the well-being of all students? • What are our current and past stories that reveal our positive core?	Attending skills • Curiosity • Mindful wonderment • Consultation • Collaboration • Strengths-based, ecological perspective • Dialogical and narrative/storied • Multicultural • Developmental
Relational Dialogue (4-R) Understanding each other's dreams. Engaged Inquiry (PIP) Considering possible actions	Steps 2, 3, 4, 5	Envision action or program potential for positive impact upon students. Possibilities about what we can do together. Dreaming with others. Dialogue with others. Past, future.	What is one small step we can take? • What are our strengths? • What others have done effectively? Elsewhere? • Where did we come from? • What are some possible directions we could take to promote student well-being and success? • What's one thing? Or the first step?	Attending skills • Curiosity • Consultation • Possibility dialogues • Strengths-based, ecological perspective • Dialogical and narrative/storied • Focus groups • Needs assessments

	Steps	Description	Questions	Skills
Relational Action (4-R) / Collaborative Action (PIP) / Meaning making	Steps 4, 5, 6	Refine propositions and action plans for enacting meaningful, life-enhancing strategies, processes, decisions, and activities. Dialogue with others. Past, present, future. Appreciation and encouragement.	• Who is participating? Who is responsible for what? • What are we (am I) going to do? What are our (my) goal(s)? • What is the first step I will take? We will take? How will we know if we are successful? Measures? • How will we assess and share our results?	Appreciation • Consultation • Strengths-based, ecological perspective • Dialogical and narrative/storied
Relational Assessment (4-R) / Action toward Community / Assessment and Reflection (PIP)	Steps 6, 7, 8, 9	Take action, gather data. Assess data. Share results: presentations, publications, etc. Acting with others. Celebrating learning power. Present, future.	• What happened? • What did we learn? • What recommendations or future action do we recommend? Next steps? • Where are we going? • How do we celebrate?	Attending skills • Curiosity • Consultation • Strengths-based, ecological perspective • Dialogical and narrative/storied
Continuous Improvement / Evolving flow, life shimmers. / Vital engagement	Step 9	Celebrate what was achieved. Celebrate process as generating learning power. Reflect on next steps and continuous improvement. Past, present, future.	• How does this build upon our best traditions? • What can we celebrate? • What other, more beautiful pathways could we build or create to make this a better place?	Attending skills • Consultation • Strengths-based, ecological perspective • Dialogical and narrative/storied • Presentations, papers, articles, etc.

* Csikszentmihalyi and Nakamura use the term "vital engagement" to show that every path is unique and offers people the opportunity to experience moments of flow (enjoyed absorption) doing what they are focused on completing, achieving, or learning. "Vital engagement" is another way of saying that the work and action have enabled us to enact "love made visible" (see Haidt, 2006, p. 224).

Appendix D
Data Templates

Table D.1 School Demographic Data: Faculty, Staff, and Administration

Population	Year	Year	Year
Faculty	#	#	#
Racial/Ethnic/Cultural Identification	Number and Percentage #/ %	#/%	#/%
Asian/Pacific Islander-American			
African-American			
Latino-American			
European-American			
Native-American			
Other			
Staff	#	#	#
Racial/Ethnic/Cultural Identification	Number and Percentage #/ %	#/%	#/%
Asian/Pacific Islander-American			
African-American			
Latino-American			
European-American			
Native-American			
Other			
Administration	#	#	#
Racial/Ethnic/Cultural Identification	Number and Percentage #/ %	#/%	#/%
Asian/Pacific Islander-American			
African-American			
Latino-American			
European-American			
Native-American			
Other			

Table D.2 School Demographic Data: Students

Population	Year	Year	Year
All Students	#	#	#
Racial/Ethnic/Cultural Identification	Number and Percentage #/ %	#/%	#/%
Asian/Pacific Islander-American African-American Latino-American European-American Native-American Other *Services*			
Special Needs/Students with Disabilities Students Designated as Disadvantaged English as a Second Language Gifted and Talented			

Table D.3 Students Meeting College Eligibility Index *

Population	Year	Year	Year
All Students	Number and Percentage #/ %	#/%	#/%
Racial/Ethnic/Cultural Identification			
Asian/Pacific Islander-American African-American Latino-American European-American Native-American Other Special Needs/Students with Disabilities Students Designated as Disadvantaged English as a Second Language			

* i.e. CSU and UC admission requirements; Middle school, ninth grade Algebra.

Table D.4 Students Enrolled in College Eligibility Index Courses *

Population	Year	Year	Year
All Students	*Number and Percentage* #/ %	#/%	#/%
Racial/Ethnic/Cultural Identification			
Asian/Pacific Islander-American African-American Latino-American European-American Native-American Other Special Needs/Students with Disabilities Students Designated as Disadvantaged English as a Second Language			

* i.e. CSU and UC admission requirements; Middle school, ninth grade Algebra.

Table D.5 High School Graduation Rate (Promotion Rates for Middle to High School or Eighth Grade Class GPA)

Population	Year	Year	Year
All Students	*Number and Percentage* #/ %	#/%	#/%
Racial/Ethnic/Cultural Identification			
Asian/Pacific Islander-American African-American Latino-American European-American Native-American Other Special Needs/Students with Disabilities Students Designated as Disadvantaged English as a Second Language			

Table D.6 Dropout/Transfer to Alternative Program Data

Population	Year	Year	Year
All Students	*Number and Percentage* #/ %	#/%	#/%
Racial/Ethnic/Cultural Identification			
Asian/Pacific Islander-American			
African-American			
Latino-American			
European-American			
Native-American			
Other			
Special Needs/Students with Disabilities			
Students Designated as Disadvantaged			
English as a Second Language			

Table D.7 Attendance (Reported Average Daily Attendance)

Population	Year	Year	Year
All Students	*Percentage* %	%	%
Racial/Ethnic/Cultural Identification			
Asian/Pacific Islander-American			
African-American			
Latino-American			
European-American			
Native-American			
Other			
Special Needs/Students with Disabilities			
Students Designated as Disadvantaged			
English as a Second Language			

Table D.8 Special Needs/Students with Disabilities Data

	Year		Year		Year	
	#	%	#	%	#	%
Asian/Pacific Islander-American						
African-American						
Latino-American						
European-American						
Native-American						
Other						
Students Designated as Disadvantaged						
English as a Second Language						

Table D.9 Safe Campus Data

	Year		Year		Year	
	#	%	#	%	#	%
Reported Fights/Offences						
Offences Against Students						
Offences Against Staff						
Sexual Harassment						
Racial Harassment						
Alcohol, Tobacco, Drug Violations						
Disruptive Behavior						
Technology/Cyberbullying						
Other						
Student Detentions						
Student Suspensions						
Student Attendance Review Board (SARB) Meetings						
Student Expulsions						

Table D.10 Participation, Contribution, and Connection In and Beyond School
Community

	Year		Year		Year	
	#	%	#	%	#	%
Extracurricular Activities						
Students Participating in Athletics						
• Football						
• Basketball						
• Baseball/Softball						
• Soccer						
• Swimming						
• Field Hockey						
Drama/performances						
Music/Chorus						
Newspaper						
Yearbook						
Clubs (how many?)						
Apprenticeships						
Regional Occupational Programs (ROP)/Job Training						
Service Projects						
Science/STEM Fairs/Activities						
Art Competitions, Fairs/Activities						
Music Competitions/Performances						
School/ Family/ Community Partnerships						
Career Fairs/Nights						
Parent/College Information Nights						
Special Topic Evenings						

Table D.11 School Achievement Data (Academic Performance Index (API) and
Standardized Results)

School	*Year*	*Year*	*Year*
School API/Target			
Racial/Ethnic/Cultural Identification	*Standardized Test Scores*	*Standardized Test Scores*	*Standardized Test Scores*
Asian/Pacific Islander-American			
African-American			
Latino-American			
European-American			
Native-American			
Other			
Special Needs/Students with Disabilities			
Students Designated as Disadvantaged			
English as a Second Language			

Table D.12 School Achievement Data (Academic Performance Index (API) and Standardized Test Results): Math

School	*Year*	*Year*	*Year*
School API/Target			
Racial/Ethnic/Cultural Identification	*Standardized Test Scores (STAR)*	*Standardized Test Scores (STAR)*	*Standardized Test Scores (STAR)*
Asian/Pacific Islander-American			
African-American			
Latino-American			
European-American			
Native-American			
Other			
Special Needs/Students with Disabilities			
Students Designated as Disadvantaged			
English as a Second Language			

Table D.13 School Achievement Data (Academic Performance Index (API) and Standardized Test Results): Reading

School	*Year*	*Year*	*Year*
School API/Target			
Racial/Ethnic/Cultural Identification	*Standardized Test Scores (STAR)*	*Standardized Test Scores (STAR)*	*Standardized Test Scores (STAR)*
Asian/Pacific Islander-American			
African-American			
Latino-American			
European-American			
Native-American			
Other			
Special Needs/Students with Disabilities			
Students Designated as Disadvantaged			
English as a Second Language			

Table D.14 School Achievement Data (Academic Performance Index (API) and Standardized Results): Other Courses

School	Year	Year	Year
School API/Target			
Racial/Ethnic/Cultural Identification	Standard-ized Test Scores	Standard-ized Test Scores	Standard-ized Test Scores
Asian/Pacific Islander-American			
African-American			
Latino-American			
European-American			
Native-American			
Other			
Special Needs/Students with Disabilities			
Students Designated as Disadvantaged			
English as a Second Language			

Table D.15 School Achievement Data (Academic Performance Index (API) and Standardized Results): Other Courses

School	Year	Year	Year
Score/Target	API	API	API
Racial/Ethnic/Cultural Identification	Standard-ized Test Scores	Standard-ized Test Scores	Standard-ized Test Scores
Asian/Pacific Islander-American			
African-American			
Latino-American			
European-American			
Native-American			
Other			
Special Needs/Students with Disabilities			
Students Designated as Disadvantaged			
English as a Second Language			

Table D.16 School Achievement Data (Academic Performance Index (API) and Standardized Results): Other Courses

School	Year	Year	Year
School API/Target			
Racial/Ethnic/Cultural Identification	*Standard-ized Test Scores*	*Standard-ized Test Scores*	*Standard-ized Test Scores*
Asian/Pacific Islander-American			
African-American			
Latino-American			
European-American			
Native-American			
Other			
Special Needs/Students with Disabilities			
Students Designated as Disadvantaged			
English as a Second Language			

Table D.17 SAT Mean Score Data

School	Year	Year	Year
Mean			
Racial/Ethnic/Cultural Identification			
Asian/Pacific Islander-American			
African-American			
Latino-American			
European-American			
Native-American			
Other			
Special Needs/Students with Disabilities			
Students Designated as Disadvantaged			
English as a Second Language			

Table D.18 ACT Mean Score Data

School	Year	Year	Year
Mean			
Racial/Ethnic/Cultural Identification			
Asian/Pacific Islander-American			
African-American			
Latino-American			
European-American			
Native-American			
Other			
Special Needs/Students with Disabilities			
Students Designated as Disadvantaged			
English as a Second Language			

Appendix E

Core Needs Assessments

1. Student Core Needs Assessment
2. Parent Core Needs Assessment
3. Teacher Core Needs Assessment
4. Administrator Core Needs Assessment
5. Support Staff Core Needs Assessment

The school counseling program is designed to help me develop my abilities in the following areas: academic, personal/social, career, and contributing to the school or greater community.

Table E.1 Student Core Concerns Needs Assessment 1: Focus on School Counseling Program

School Counseling Program: *School counselors and the school counseling program help me to develop my abilities in:*	Strongly Disagree	Disagree	Agree	Strongly Agree
	1	2	3	4
a. Academic and elective courses; in learning to see myself as always learning.	1	2	3	4
b. Personal social relationships; in learning how to work effectively and respectfully with many different types of people.	1	2	3	4
c. Career aspirations; in learning about different career, college, and post-secondary pathways that are possible.	1	2	3	4
d. Contributions to school and community; learning about ways I can participate in school activities, such as athletics, theater, music, community service activities, etc.	1	2	3	4
e. Promoting my own sense of wellness and well-being	1	2	3	4

continued

Table E.1 continued

School Program and Focus:	Strongly Disagree 1	Disagree 2	Agree 3	Strongly Agree 4
The school counselor or school counseling program has helped me look at my own strengths.	1	2	3	4
The school counselor or school counseling program keeps me informed about activities and resources, such as tutoring, AVID, PUENTE, etc.	1	2	3	4
My experience at school is oriented to build on my strengths and what I am doing right or well in class, at home, and in the community.	1	2	3	4
The school counselor program provides information, data, and other materials to show how the school counseling program is designed to help all students live up to their potential.	1	2	3	4
I feel the school counselors are there to stand up for me and to help me live up to my potential as a student and as a participant and contributor to our school and greater community.	1	2	3	4
There is at least one person at school who I can talk to and who will support me if I have a problem or am stuck in a bad situation.	1	2	3	4
School counselors really help promote a peaceful and connected school community.	1	2	3	4
I feel confident in myself as a learner or have one area where I feel I am developing competence and mastery.	1	2	3	4

My favorite class is_____ [no teacher names]

One thing that I think is really great about this school is:

_____

_____

One thing that would make this school a stronger learning community is:

_____

_____

The school counseling program is designed to help students develop their abilities in the following areas: academic, personal/social, career, and contributing to the school or greater community.

Table E.2 Parent Core Concerns Needs Assessment 2: Focus on School Counseling Program

School Counseling Program: School counselors and the school counseling program help my student(s) to develop his/her abilities in:	Strongly Disagree 1	Disagree 2	Agree 3	Strongly Agree 4
a. Academic and elective courses; helping students to see themselves as capable learners or directing them to resources, such as tutoring, etc.	1	2	3	4
b. Personal social relationships; helping students to learn how to work effectively and respectfully with many different types of people, such as listening and responding to others.	1	2	3	4
c. Career aspirations; in learning about different career, college, and post-secondary pathways. Providing college or career nights where parents can receive information.	1	2	3	4
d. Contributions to school and community; learning about ways students can participate in school activities, such as athletics, theater, music, community service activities, etc. Parents receive current information about positive activities at school and the community.	1	2	3	4
e. Promoting students' own sense of wellness and well-being.	1	2	3	4
School Program and Focus:				
You have received materials that have informed you about the school counseling program's vision or mission.	1	2	3	4
You have received a disclosure statement regarding your child's school counselor's education, training, and orientation.	1	2	3	4
Your student's experience at school is oriented to build on their strengths and what they are doing right or well in class, at home, and in the community.	1	2	3	4

continued

Table E.2 continued

School Program and Focus:	Strongly Disagree 1	Disagree 2	Agree 3	Strongly Agree 4
The school counselor program provides information, data, and other materials to show how the school counseling program is designed to help all students live up to their potential. The school counselor or school counseling program keeps me informed about activities and resources, such as tutoring, AVID, PUENTE, etc.	1	2	3	4
I feel the school counselors are there to advocate for my child and to help them live up to their potential as learners and as participants and contributors at school and as citizens in the greater community.	1	2	3	4
There is at least one person at school who your child can talk to and who will support them if they have a problem or are stuck in a bad situation.	1	2	3	4
There is at least one person at school who I can talk to and who will support me if my child has a problem or I feel my child is stuck in a bad situation.	1	2	3	4
School counselors really help promote a peaceful and connected school community.	1	2	3	4
I feel confident in my child as a learner who has at least one area where they feel they are developing competence and mastery.	1	2	3	4

My student's favorite class is_____ [no teacher names]

One thing that I think is really great about this school is:

_____

_____

One thing that would make this school a stronger learning community is:

_____

_____

The school counseling program is designed to help students develop their abilities in the following areas: academic, personal/social, career, and contributing to the school or greater community.

Table E.3 Teacher Core Concerns Needs Assessment 3: Focus on School Counseling Program

School Counseling Program: School counselors and the school counseling program collaborate with teachers and support students to develop their abilities in:	Strongly Disagree	Disagree	Agree	Strongly Agree
	1	2	3	4
a. Academic and elective courses; helping students to see themselves as capable learners or directing them to resources, such as tutoring, etc.	1	2	3	4
b. Personal social relationships; helping students to learn how to work effectively and respectfully with many different types of people, such as listening and responding to others.	1	2	3	4
c. Career aspirations; in learning about different career, college, and post-secondary requirements. Providing materials to both students and teachers.	1	2	3	4
d. Contributions to school and community; learning about ways students can participate in school activities, such as athletics, theater, music, community service activities, etc. Teachers receive current information about positive activities at school and the community.	1	2	3	4
e. Promoting students' own sense of wellness and well-being.	1	2	3	4

School Program and Focus:

You have received materials that have informed you about the school counseling program's vision or mission.	1	2	3	4
You have received a disclosure statement regarding each school counselor's education, training, and orientation.	1	2	3	4
You have been informed of the school counselor's orientation to build on student strengths.	1	2	3	4

continued

Table E.3 continued

School Program and Focus:	Strongly Disagree 1	Disagree 2	Agree 3	Strongly Agree 4
The school counselor program provides information, data, and other materials to show how the school counseling program is designed to collaborate with teachers to help all students live up to their potential, using guidance lessons, activities, and resources, such as tutoring, AVID, PUENTE, etc.	1	2	3	4
I feel the school counselors are there to advocate for children and to help them live up to their potential as learners.	1	2	3	4
I try to be a person at school who students can talk to; I try to support them and have them work with their counselor if they have a problem or are stuck in a bad situation.	1	2	3	4
I believe that all students can and are capable of learning, even if it is learning that they do not like school.	1	2	3	4
School counselors really help promote a peaceful and connected school community.	1	2	3	4
I feel confident that the school counselors are delivering a school counseling program that serves the school well.	1	2	3	4

One thing I really like about this school in the past or currently is:

_____

_____

One thing that would make this school a stronger learning community is:

_____

_____

One thing that would make the school counseling program better is:

_____

_____

The school counseling program is designed to help students develop their abilities in the following areas: academic, personal/social, career, and contributing to the school or greater community.

Table E.4 Administrator Core Concerns Needs Assessment 4: Focus on School Counseling Program

School Counseling Program: School counselors and the school counseling program collaborate with teachers and support students to develop their abilities in:	Strongly Disagree	Disagree	Agree	Strongly Agree
	1	2	3	4
a. Academic and elective courses; helping students to see themselves as capable learners or directing them to resources, such as tutoring, etc.	1	2	3	4
b. Personal social relationships; helping students to learn how to work effectively and respectfully with many different types of people, such as listening and responding to others.	1	2	3	4
c. Career aspirations; in learning about different career, college, and post-secondary requirements. Providing materials to both students and teachers.	1	2	3	4
d. Contributions to school and community; learning about ways students can participate in school activities, such as athletics, theater, music, community service activities, etc. Teachers receive current information about positive activities at school and the community.	1	2	3	4
e. Promoting students' own sense of wellness and well-being.	1	2	3	4
School Program and Focus:				
You have received materials that have informed you about the school counseling program's vision or mission.	1	2	3	4
The school counseling program is strongly aligned with the American School Counselor Association (ASCA) National Model	1	2	3	4

continued

Table E.4 continued

School Program and Focus:	Strongly Disagree 1	Disagree 2	Agree 3	Strongly Agree 4
There is an annually reviewed Crisis Management Plan in place; school counselors have psychologist roles.	1	2	3	4
The school counselor program provides information, data, and other materials to show how the school counseling program is designed to collaborate with teachers to help all students live up to their potential, using guidance lessons, activities, and resources, such as tutoring, AVID, PUENTE, etc.	1	2	3	4
The school counselor role is to advocate for children and to help them live up to their potential as learners.	1	2	3	4
You have been informed of the school counselor's orientation to build on student strengths.	1	2	3	4
The school counseling program tracks data over three-year periods and defines their vision, mission, and goals around existing data.	1	2	3	4
School counselors really help promote a peaceful and connected school community.	1	2	3	4
I feel confident that the school counselors are delivering a school counseling program that serves the school well.	1	2	3	4

One thing I really like about this school in the past or currently is:

_____

_____

One thing that would make this school a stronger learning community is:

_____

_____

One thing that would make the school counseling program better is:

_____

_____

The school counseling program is designed to help students develop their abilities in the following areas: academic, personal/social, career, and contributing to the school or greater community.

Table E.5 Support Staff Core Concerns Needs Assessment 5: Focus on School Counseling Program

School Counseling Program: School counselors and the school counseling program collaborate with teachers and support students to develop their abilities in:	Strongly Disagree	Disagree	Agree	Strongly Agree
	1	2	3	4
a. Academic and elective courses; helping students to see themselves as capable learners or directing them to resources, such as tutoring, etc.	1	2	3	4
b. Personal social relationships; helping students to learn how to work effectively and respectfully with many different types of people, such as listening and responding to others.	1	2	3	4
c. Career aspirations; in learning about different career, college, and post-secondary requirements. Providing materials to both students and teachers.	1	2	3	4
d. Contributions to school and community; learning about ways students can participate in school activities, such as athletics, theater, music, community service activities, etc. Teachers receive current information about positive activities at school and the community.	1	2	3	4
e. Promoting students' own sense of wellness and well-being.	1	2	3	4

School Program and Focus:

You have received materials that have informed you about the school counseling program's vision or mission in helping all children.	1	2	3	4
You have received a disclosure statement regarding the school counselors' education, training, orientation, and ethical obligation to be confidential about what students share.	1	2	3	4

continued

Table E.5 continued

School Program and Focus:	Strongly Disagree 1	Disagree 2	Agree 3	Strongly Agree 4
You see that the school counseling program is oriented to build on students' strengths and what they are doing right or well in class, at home, and in the community.	1	2	3	4
The school counselor program provides information, data, and other materials to show how the school counseling program is designed to help all students live up to their potential. The school counselor or school counseling program keeps support staff informed about activities and resources, such as tutoring, AVID, PUENTE, etc.	1	2	3	4
I feel the school counselors are there to advocate for children and to help them live up to their potential as learners and as participants and contributors at school and as citizens in the greater community.	1	2	3	4
I try to be a person at school who students can talk to and I [or you] support students if they have a problem or are stuck in a bad situation by referring them to the school counselor.	1	2	3	4
This is a school where all kids can find at least one person who they can talk to and who will support them if they have a problem or feel stuck in a bad situation.	1	2	3	4
School counselors really help promote a peaceful and connected school community.	1	2	3	4
I have a lot of faith in kids as learners; the students I know have at least one area where they feel they are developing competence and mastery.	1	2	3	4

One thing I really like about this school in the past or currently is:

_____

_____

One thing that would make this school a stronger learning community is:

_____

_____

One thing that would make the school counseling program better is:

_____

_____

Appendix F
Generic Parent Permission Form

PARENT PERMISSION FORM FOR _____

Dear Parent/Guardian,

_____ School District, in cooperation with the Master's in School Counseling Program at California State University, East Bay, is providing freshmen students with the _____ Guidance Curriculum in freshmen Health classes. The _____ Guidance Curriculum, in accordance with the Health curriculum, will focus on high school graduation readiness and requirements, college readiness information, and high school transition skills. The guidance curriculum will be implemented by_____, candidates for a Master's Degree in School Counseling at California State University, East Bay.

If you consent for your child to participate in this guidance curriculum, the following will occur:

- Your child will be asked to participate in the _____ Guidance Curriculum including individual writings and group activities.
- This will take place once a month in their regular Health classroom as part of the scheduled curriculum.
- Your child will turn in all written and group assignments and these will be returned to them at the end of the 20___–20___ school year. Data will be collected in the form of surveys and questionnaires, and student anonymity and confidentiality will be respected. The benefits for students participating in the _____ Guidance Curriculum are not limited to but include high school graduation readiness and requirements, college readiness information, decision making skills, team building skills, and social skills development. The risks for students participating in the curriculum may be increased awareness of the difficulty in completing the required coursework for high school graduation and college preparedness. There will be no cost for participating in the curriculum nor any compensation for the student's

participation. _____ are currently working as volunteer, counselors-in-training at _____School under the supervision of credentialed counselors _____ and _____. If you have any questions or concerns, please contact _____ at (000) 000–0000 ext. 001, _____ at (000) 000–0000 ext. 02, or the Principal of _____School, _____ at (000) 000–0000 ext. 03. _

Please fill out this form to acknowledge if your child will participate. The form can be returned to your child's Health teacher.

Parent Acknowledgement for Student Participation:

My son/daughter, _____ has permission to participate in the _____ Guidance Curriculum, held by _____ the freshmen support counseling interns at _____ High School.

_____

Parent/Guardian Signature

_____

Date

Student Acknowledgement for Participation:

I agree to participate in the _____Guidance Curriculum held by _____. I understand that I have the right to pass and advocate for my learning.

_____

Student Signature

_____

Date

Appendix G
Mapping the Driving and Restraining Forces (MDRF)

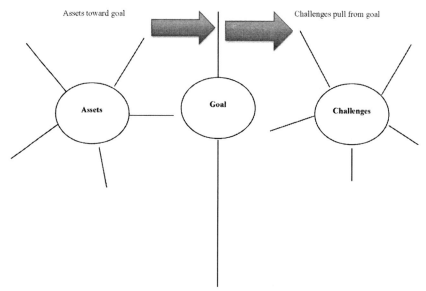

Please use the basic template to map out the assets or forces supporting moving toward the goal and the challenges or forces pulling back from movement toward the goal.

Figure G.1 Mapping the Driving and Restraining Forces (MDRF) Worksheet: Forces for Change, Forces against Change.

Appendix H
Focus Group, Fishbowl Story Group, and Video Story Focus Group Guidelines
Roles, Skills, Participation, and Agreements

These guidelines will talk about three basic focus groups: 1) Focus Groups that can include Restorative Justice Circles, Talking Circles, Story Circles, Focus Story Groups, and other such names; 2) Fishbowl Story Groups and Bearing Witness Circles are similar to the focus groups, only they have observers or individuals bearing witness to what those in the focus group are saying; 3) Video Story Focus Groups are focus groups that are recorded and edited to provide adults and those in power who are "unable to attend" a fishbowl group a way to see and hear what the focus group wants them to hear.

Basic Focus Group Requirements

1. *Helping Professional/Participatory Leader* defines or takes role as focus group *Facilitator*. The facilitator is frequently a counselor, a professional-in-training, or another helping professional with experience leading groups, listening well, fostering rapport, etc. The facilitator should have no power (giving a grade or having authority to punish) over the group participants; the facilitator cannot be a school administrator or other school community member who is viewed as an enforcer of rules; it is best to have a helping professional, student advocate, or otherwise neutral party act as facilitator.
2. Facilitator talks to department leader and/or *site administrator* about facilitating a focus group.
   a. Discusses goal, i.e., finding out level of care and support, high expectations, or meaningful participation perceived by participants.
      i.   If possible, recommend and/or take actions to address recommendations emerging from the group.
   b. Discusses permission and permission form; confidentiality, invitations to participate, secure location for focus group, and district (if required) approval.
3. *Facilitator skills*. Listen, listen, listen. Enter the world of those in the group as much as possible. Empathize with observers. Make sure that

those venting about frustrations or problems do not use names. Some of the counseling core skills used are:

   a. *attending skills*: listening, empathic understanding, clarification, etc. (Ivey et al., 2006);
   b. *curiosity listening*: "Why do you think that is?" "Tell me some more about" (Winslade & Monk, 2007);
   c. *mindful wonderment*: "Wow! I'm wondering what other ways you see teachers and other adults helping students." "Have you ever wondered if" (Lewis et al., 2010);
   d. *community agreements* (Gibbs, 2006) (see below).

4. *Focus Group Membership*
   a. *Facilitator*. See above.
   b. *Students*. Initially, membership should be restricted to students at the same grade level, i.e., a seventh grade group, eighth grade group, etc. The purpose of the grade-level grouping is to insure that younger students have a voice.
      i. *Cliques*. Additionally, it is important to assess the impact and power of student cliques on campus. If students seem to think there are a lot of cliques and in and out groups, it is best to initially include groups that have students (or faculty) from the same cliques; the goal is to make sure they talk and share their world, not get into conflicts. If running a series of groups with different cliques, it is important to conduct a mixed follow up with members from the different groups.
      ii. If considering a mixed group follow up, conduct a socio-gram process asking each person in the first group to name the three most influential members of the group they are in.
         – Choose members who are in high regard to participate in the mixed groups.
   c. *Recorder*. Someone should be invited to take notes to record the session. The notes should be shared with key, if not all, participants to insure that they agree the notes are accurate or suggest possible revisions.

5. *Students as Consultants and Participatory Leaders*. Invite the students to join the group planning as consultants and participatory leaders. The goal of the group is to enter and share their understanding, not to impose the adult world on their understanding. The role of the facilitator and adult planner is to function more as an anthropologist who is respectfully entering and learning about another culture than as a colonizer who is imposing a predetermined understanding upon that culture. The essential point is that the facilitators are really trying to model a belief that students are capable of making significant and positive contributions to their school if adults will set up the conditions for them to take action.

6. *Agreements.* Make sure that there are community agreements that define expected behaviors for both group participants and group observers.
7. Participants should be told to *turn off cell phones, iPads, computers,* and other *electronic devices.* The process is about speaking and listening without unnecessary interruptions.
8. The *time* should be about 45–65 minutes; less than 45 minutes can be too short, while over 65 minutes can lead to fatigue.
9. The *place* should be free from distractions, such as people entering and exiting the room, bringing hall passes, etc. Try to conduct the session in a clean room that does not have trash or distracting materials posted on the walls, too. If conducting a fishbowl focus group, make sure that the observers outside of the focus group are at least 3–5 feet back in a circle quietly observing the group.
10. The *size* of focus groups should be between six and ten, not too small and not too large, to be able to facilitate dialogue between members and to foster areas of consensus.

Basic Focus Group Structure and Process

What is the purpose and audience for the focus group? First and foremost, it is important to be clear about why a focus group is being conducted. Focus groups are powerful tools for promoting informative, reflective, and evolving conversations where all voices are heard. Focus groups are empowering for students and promoting student wellness, if what is shared in the group is used in some way to prompt changes or action toward changes. Focus groups can create space for sharing untold stories, and define safe space where truth can be spoken to power without fear of repercussions or retributions. Focus groups are opportunities for multiple voices to be heard in order to demonstrate a valuing of different readings of events. The structure of the focus groups is NOT about venting but about finding the story undergirding any frustration or anger and moving toward the positive core, and what is referred to as promoting relational possibilities found in a preferred future. Focus groups can foster a reflective space where new relational possibilities can be generated and defined. This boils down to: what can be done to make this a more connected school community that promotes the wellness of all students?

Invitation, Recruitment, Screening, and Selection

It is important to invite and recruit diverse students. The same is true for adults, but their role is generally to act as witnesses to the student conversations taking place in fishbowl focus groups. See the comments regarding membership as providing guidelines for defining how to determine who will be in the group.

Create a general announcement about the group to send to teachers, staff, administrators, and other school stakeholders. Make sure that you mention the time commitment and pre-session interest meetings. Make sure teachers have enough information to be able to encourage interested and diverse students to attend the interest meetings. The key to creating interest is to talk about the focus groups as giving voice to many students and as, hopefully, leading to positive change that helps enhance the school as a learning community.

Planning meeting. Make sure students are invited to join in a planning meeting. Invite students to become more actively engaged in figuring out what can be done to make their school a more connected learning community that promotes the wellness of all students. They are also invited to review prompts.

Assessments. You may want to use Student Core Concerns Needs Assessment 1: Focus on School Counseling Program (Appendix E) or the mapping the Driving and Restraining Forces (mDRF) Worksheet (Appendix G) during the planning meeting to help the students begin thinking about relational possibilities and their role in constructing a more vibrant school community. This is the stage where you invite them to act as student consultants and to become participatory leaders in the focus group and change process. Again, the goal is joining with students to create a process that promotes greater wellness on the school campus.

Permission. During the invitation stage and planning sessions, make sure that you get the names of the participants. Give them permission forms, which may be adapted from Appendix F. Let potential participants know how necessary permission forms are and that they are created to ensure the *respect* and *wellness* of both the participants and the parents of the participants. The facilitator lets interested students know they will get a confirmation regarding the day and time for the focus group upon receipt of the permission form.

Please note that focus groups require an additional layer of privacy protection, because the facilitator cannot guarantee that the participants of the group will not reveal each other's contributions to the group discussion once it has ended.

In addition to the warning about "loss of privacy is a potential risk" on the permission form, the informed consent should contain something like:

> Because the focus groups and talking circles include discussion of personal opinions, extra measures will be taken to protect each participant's privacy. The facilitator will begin the focus group by asking the participants to agree to the importance of keeping information discussed in the focus group confidential. She or he will then ask each participant to verbally agree to keep everything discussed in the room confidential, and will remind them at the end of the group

not to discuss the material outside. Still, there is a potential risk regarding your privacy.

If developing a recording of the session, there should be an explicit statement regarding the purposes and audience for the recording; participants should have final say over what portion of their story can be shared.

Time commitment. Students are invited to participate in the planning, pre-session, session, and post-session meetings. At the same time, as long as they have a permission slip, merely attending the focus group pre-session and session group is a sufficient commitment.

Pre-Session Interest Meeting, Assessment (15–30 Minutes)

Meet with participants and observers in separate meetings to orient them. The purpose of the pre-session is to make sure to review the agreements, emphasizing confidentiality, not using names to point out complaints, etc.

Session (30–60 Minutes)

Room and seating should be adequate for the focus group, talking circle, or entire fishbowl story group. The room should be free from distractions, such as people entering and exiting the room, bringing hall passes, etc. Name tags, drinks, and other materials are available upon entering the room.

Beginning session. The session begins with a brief introduction by the facilitator, where he/she describes his/her role and the purpose of the focus group. The facilitator invites each person in the focus group to introduce him/herself.

Agreements. The facilitator affirms agreements and that participants and observers are to *turn off phones, handheld devices, iPads, computers,* and other *electronic devices that pull your attention from listening to others.* The focus group process is about speaking and listening without unnecessary interruptions.

The facilitator talks about confidentiality and the limits of confidentiality in groups. What is said and expressed in the group should be respected as something said in confidence. It should not be talked about with others outside of the group. Note that what is talked about will be documented but that no names will be attributed to what is said; there will merely be a list of participants as part of the documentation, which will be focused on advocating for any changes recommended by the focus group or fishbowl focus group. Affirm that everyone has guiding questions for the session.

Specific agreements are reviewed (based on Gibbs, 2006); members are asked if they want to add any additional agreements; members are asked if they agree with the agreements; the facilitator should make eye contact or seek confirmation from each member to affirm that they approve of the agreements:

Participants

Attentive listening
Self-respect
Mutual respect
No put downs
Encourage all participants to speak their truth/tell their story.

Prompts. The facilitator works from a prompt list. There should be between five and seven prompts, but no more than seven prompts. Each participant is asked the same question. The facilitator rotates the questions so that a different person is asked the question the first time. After asking the participants, the facilitator uses curiosity questioning or mindful wonderment to elicit further refection and dialogue about the responses. The facilitator is aware that the goal is to move the conversation toward action during the post-session review.

Ending session. The facilitator thanks the participants. The participants are asked for any comments they have about their experience. The facilitator may ask, "What could we do to make the next focus group better?" If conducting a fishbowl, the observers are invited to thank the group and to ask questions of clarification. It is important that the questions are framed in terms of understanding and not judging. If the session has resulted in some possible directions for action, the facilitator may ask participants about pursuing some form of action during a post-session meeting.

Post-Session

The recorder offers his/her notes to key participants for their review and possible suggestions for revision. A post-session meeting is called that includes both participants. The session notes are reviewed and the facilitator attempts to define some relational possibilities that could be acted upon to take one step toward improving the school's wellness.

Proposed actions. Proposed actions come from summarizing what was learned and asking, "Now that we know these things, what specific actions can we take together to address one of our concerns?" Then, "What would be our second and third concern to be addressed?" This is where the participants are invited to take up responsibility and to join to figure out what we can do together moving shoulder to shoulder to make our school better. The language has to be inclusive and genuine. The participants should be oriented to being in a community where there are no guarantees, but that the facilitator promises to be an advocate on their behalf.

Reporting results. Because focus groups invite students into a participative process, it is important to document what has happened before, during, and after the focus group. Reports can be divided into: pre-session, session, post-session, and recommendations. Names should not be attributed to any person.

Additional Requirement for Fishbowl Focus Groups

The essential difference between a focus group and a fishbowl or bearing witness story group is that the fishbowl has a group of adults or observers sitting outside of the group bearing witness to what is being said. The process places the adults in a position where they listen to what is important to students, and where the students talking inside the circle experience greater validation and power as they speak their own truth to the adults who are showing the willingness to listen.

Adult and ally participants. The fishbowl or bearing witness story group generally invites in adult members to bear witness to the stories the youth are sharing. The adult role is to listen and not disrupt or add to the conversation within the group. It is vital that the adults understand that their job is to listen deeply and bear witness to the group members' experience.

Room and Seating

If conducting a fishbowl story group, make sure that the observers outside of the focus group are at least 3–5 feet back in a circle where they can quietly observe the group.

Beginning the Session

If conducting a fishbowl, the facilitator invites the observers to introduce themselves. Participants and observers are given copies of the story group prompts. A recorder should take notes to ensure that every voice is captured.

Fishbowl Observers Agree to:

Attentive listening
Respectful listening
No speaking or comments
Stay for entire session
If willing, offer self as ally at end of session.

Ending the Fishbowl Session

The facilitator thanks observers. If the session has resulted in some possible directions for action, the facilitator may ask participants and observers about pursuing some form of action during a post-session meeting.

Additional Requirements for Video Story Groups

The essential difference between a fishbowl focus group and a video story group is that the session is video recorded and edited in order to share what the group has explored with adults who have agreed to bear witness to what is being said. There are times when administrators "do not have time" to attend fishbowls. Recorded sessions that develop a clear student narrative in response to the prompts can be very powerful for informing administrators and others about the world and experience of a group of students at the school.

The limits of privacy are clear and should be explicit in the parent permission and student consent forms. Like the fishbowl, the process places the adults in a position where they listen to what is important to students, and where the students talking inside the circle experience greater validation and power as they speak their own truth to the adults who are showing the willingness to listen. The difference is that the students can edit the recording to make sure that the adults hear what the students want them to hear. This is because, if recording sessions, participants should have the last say over what portions of their story gets shared. The audience(s) should understand the importance of the facilitator and students shaping what is shared.

Possible Prompts for Initial Focus Group

1. What is it that gives the most life and sense of positive wellness or well-being to you when you are at school?
2. How are adults helping you develop a sense of your own learning power? How do adults show their belief in you as a learner or as someone who is capable of making positive contributions to the school community?
3. How well does the school teach and how well do the adults in school model interpersonal communication? That is, listening, speaking, responding respectfully and directly.
4. In your classes and at school, talk about the choices you get to make and sense of control you have in specific situations. Briefly talk about how you have learned or are learning basic decision making skills and even an appreciation for the complexity of the decision making process.
5. To you, what is the most meaningful thing you do at school, be it working toward a specific goal, learning something new, or even making sense of your own life?
6. If you were to make recommendations for helping this school become a better place for all students, what specific recommendations would you make?
7. If you were asked to make recommendations about how adults could support and care for students, what specific recommendations would you offer?

Possible Follow-Up Focus Group Prompts

Please share a summary of the previous focus group recommendations with these prompts.

1. What changes have you witnessed at school or in yourself as the result of the change efforts over the past few/three months? Do you feel more life and a sense of positive wellness or well-being when you are at school?

2. How are adults helping you develop a sense of your own learning power? How are adults showing their belief in you as a learner or as someone who is capable of making positive contributions to the school community?

3. Do you have any examples of how adults in school are modeling interpersonal communication? That is, listening, speaking, responding respectfully and directly.

4. In your classes and at school, talk about the choices you get to make and sense of control you have in specific situations. Briefly talk about how you are learning basic decision making skills and even an appreciation for the complexity of the decision making process.

5. To you, what is the most meaningful thing you have done at school in the past few/three months, be it working toward a specific goal, learning something new, or even making sense of your own life?

6. How have the student recommendations for helping this school become a better place for all students been fulfilled? What specific recommendations would you make right now?

7. Given the specific recommendations about how adults could support and care for students, what specific additional recommendations would you offer?

Appendix I
PIP and AI Action Worksheet

Table I.1 PIP and AI Action Worksheet

Inquiry and Action Steps	Key Questions	Reflections/Actions
Open Inquiry **PIP Phase 1: Initiating Conversations and Identifying Challenges** **AI Phase 1: Relational Connection** Conversations have taken place with individuals, small groups, and perhaps even the entire school. You have a sense of different perspectives and possibilities.	1) What do I see? What do you see? What do we see? What do we see working for students? How do we know? Who is benefiting, perhaps "blossoming", in our school environment—MORE importantly, who is not? 2) What do I see and hear? What do you see and hear? What do "we" as a group or community see and hear? 3) Have we included diverse voices? Including "diverse voices" should not be the fourth question to be considered—it's the voices that are not being heard that we, as advocates, are after. 4) How do we engage the voices of students and families who are not experiencing success?	
Focused Inquiry **PIP Phase 2: Engaged Inquiry** **AI Phase 1: Relational Dialogue** Conversations continue. The inquiry begins to look for and to share data that	1) What are our narratives? Preferred narrative? 2) What do students, families, teachers, etc. have to say about their school experience? 3) What is our positive core? What practices demonstrate our commitment to students? 4) What if . . .? What might we do to better serve students?	

continued

Table I.1 continued

Inquiry and Action Steps	Key Questions	Reflections/Actions
might inform the conversations. The inquiry becomes more focused and moves toward defining possible actions.	5) Questions are explored with mindful wonder. 6) What would happen if we tried . . .? 7) What are some possible courses of action?	
Focused Inquiry **PIP Phase 2: Engaged Inquiry** **PIP Phase 3: Collaborative Action** **AI Phase 1: Relational Dialogue** **AI Phase 3: Relational Action** **Choosing a strategy or action plan.** **Action plan defines that clear, concrete, specific, and measurable goal(s) are defined:** *Clear*: You can see your goal(s) and you have an action plan pathway for getting to the goal(s). *Concrete*: You can measure each step toward the goal. *Specific*: You have targeted a specific group, grade level, or problem.	1) What problem(s) or challenge(s) do we want to address? 2) What data do you have to inform an action plan and goal(s)? 3) How do you propose to implement your action plan? 4) What are the assumptions underlying the proposed strategy or action? 5) How is your action plan meaningful, measurable, and realistic in terms of goal(s)?	
Meaningfulness a) counselors, b) teachers, c) administrators, d) students, e) parents and other stakeholders support the goal as important to school. You have allies.	1) Who finds the goal meaningful? 2) How have students, teachers, families, etc. defined this action plan? 3) Who will be an ally in your efforts?	

continued

Table I.1 continued

Inquiry and Action Steps	Key Questions	Reflections/Actions
Measureable You have decided what you are going to assess or measure to determine progress or results.	1) How will you measure the effectiveness of the strategy? 2) How will you know you reach or do not reach your goal? 3) In other words, how will you know when you get there?	
Realistic You (as a group) are clear about being able to achieve the goal. The time allotted and systemic barriers can be managed. For instance, you decide to develop a SPARC as a first step and baseline for transforming your program.	1) How realistic is the action plan within the time frame? 2) Should you break the action plan into something shorter and more attainable?	
Time Frame and Limits The goal(s) we decided upon can be attained in the time we (as a group) have budgeted for it.	1) What is our time frame? 2) What are the limits on the time of the team?	
Analysis and Reflection: Impact of the actions PIP Phase 4: Community Assessment **AI Phase 4: Relational Assessment and Reflection** We have committed to sharing the impact of our actions by blocking time to analyze and document our outcomes.	1) How are we going to analyze and share the impact of our actions?	
Dialogue and Alignment with Stories in Ecosystem We have studied and assessed how our actions might be aligned with school, district, and community values, hopes, dreams, and stories.	1) Where do our goals and actions fit in the bigger story of the school, district, and community? 2) Who do we talk to about what we have done? 3) Where is a community of practice that we can share our work with?	

Appendix J
Outline for Writing Action Research Paper Using the Participatory Inquiry Process (PIP)

The purpose of this outline is to guide your work and to enable other future researchers to replicate your work in their own settings. You are developing a map for others to follow and to understand your context, your process, your actions, and your results.

1. *Introduction*
   1.1 Problem statement or challenge being addressed
   1.2 Ecological context
       1.2.1 Community
           1.2.1.1 Size and location of city
       1.2.2 School
           1.2.2.1 Size and location of school
   1.3 Research question(s)—What do you wonder? What challenge are you going to address? Who are your collaborators in your lifescaping or future forming effort? What outcomes do you hope your actions will achieve. What do you envision?
   1.4 Summary description of PIP and the intervention
2. *Literature Review* (2–3 pages)
   2.1 Relevant literature that you have reviewed
   2.2 The particular perspective that you will use in your PIP action research.
3. *Community, School, Study Sample* (Students)
   3.1 Your community
       3.1.1 Demographic data: race, income level, educational level (if possible)
   3.2 Your school
       3.2.1 Demographic data: race, test scores by race, education level of parents, college eligibility index by race
   3.3 Study sample, i.e., with whom will you conduct your intervention/ evaluation
       3.3.1 Grade level
       3.3.2 Number of students (subjects), racial background, etc.

4. *Methodology*
   4.1 Action Research Using the Participatory Inquiry Process (PIP)
   4.2 PIP's Four Phases and Nine Steps
5. *Phase 1: Initiating Conversations and Identifying Challenges*
   5.1 *Step 1.* Professionals-in-training begin the inquiry process by looking at the school environment, accessible school data, and other school-wide sources of information that will begin to provide the school's narrative (see PIP Phases and Steps).
      5.1.1 Professionals-in-training enter the community like an anthropologist by listening to individuals and groups to hear some of the school's stories and story elements.
      5.1.2 What are the school's strengths, assets, and perceived challenges as a learning community? Collaboratively begin to define a lifescaping challenge to be addressed, typically a student group being under-served.
      5.1.3 Examine challenges and aspirations to put forward possibility pathways for solving a problem based on data that impacts the delivery of student services or the school's lifescape as a learning community.
   5.2 *Step 2.* Conversations and collaborations take place among site supervisors, professionals-in-training, school counselors, school psychologists, teachers, administrators, students, parents, and other stakeholders.
      5.2.1 Conversations are directed toward success stories in the past, outstanding practices and traditions, possible futures, ways to transform practices, and a best possible and dreamed for lifescape for promoting positive student outcomes.
6. *Phase 2: Engaged Inquiry*
   6.1 *Step 3.* Using engaged inquiry, professional resources, responses, and possibilities for solutions to developing the learning lifescape are researched.
      6.1.1 Resources within the school community are assessed and reflected on in framing how to address the challenge.
         6.1.1.1 What resources, services, and strategies are currently in place to serve students?
         6.1.1.2 What's working? What's not?
         6.1.1.3 What areas could be initiated, expanded, or improved?
   6.2 *Step 4.* Using available school-based data, baseline, comparative, and data trends are investigated and reflected upon by the learning community stakeholders or those engaged in the PIP.
      6.2.1 Additional data are collected from teachers, parents, students and other stakeholders.
         6.2.1.1 Qualitative and quantitative data is gathered through surveys, focus groups, meetings,

interviews, school walk-throughs and program observations.

6.2.1.2 Professionals-in-training may lead the learning community to consider the learning lifescape:

6.2.1.2.1 What questions should be posed about the data?

6.2.1.2.2 What do we hope to learn?

6.2.1.2.3 What data sources will you use?

6.2.1.2.4 What procedures will you use to collect or obtain data?

6.2.1.2.5 Develop a plan to implement Phase 3.

7. *Phase 3: Collaborative Action*

7.1 *Step 5.* Conversations about problems, challenges, and actions are directed toward defining meaningful, measurable, and realistic goals that address the concern. A choice is made regarding what action(s) to take to change the learning lifescape.

7.1.1 Describe your intervention in detail.

7.1.2 Form a problem statement, challenge statement or lifescaping statement.

7.1.3 Form a hypothesis.

7.1.3.1 What will change?

7.1.3.2 How will you measure the change?

7.1.4 *Step 6.* Actions are taken to put the agreed upon strategy(s) into practice.

7.1.4.1 Document challenges, adjustments, and successes in the actions.

8. *Phase 4: Community Assessment and Reflection*

8.1 *Step 7.* Lifescaping actions are evaluated and results discussed with the learning community.

8.1.1 Data Collection—describe data collection in detail (so that someone else could do it if you went on vacation, won the lottery and ran away, etc.)

8.1.1.1 How will you collect the data?

8.1.1.2 Data analysis—how will you analyze and present each type of data that you collect?

8.1.1.3 Results—were the results consistent with what the literature predicted?

8.1.1.4 Were the results what you anticipated?

8.1.1.5 What are the implications for your school or the students?

8.1.2 *Limitations*—what are the limitations to your study? Were there roadblocks or other unanticipated variables that impacted your study?

8.1.3 *Reflection*—actions are reflected upon and efforts are shared, e.g. with students in the school, department members, school community, school board, college or university class, etc.

    8.1.3.1   Feedback from stakeholders and interested parties is reflected on and used, if possible.

8.2 *Step 8.* The strategy is adapted accordingly via learning community reflection. What would you do differently?

    8.2.1 Recommendations—what are the implications for additional research, i.e., what type of additional research should follow up on the results of your study?

8.3 *Step 9.* Talk about any action you plan to take to put the revised strategy into practice.

    8.3.1 Define a time frame to revisit what has been done and the strategy being implemented. Like expiration dates on milk cartons, a time is set in order to revisit, reassess, revise, and renew practice.

    8.3.2 How do you build on or maintain your PIP lifescaping efforts?

9. *Conclusion* (half page).

Appendix K
Write Way Support Materials

Guidance Curriculum Action Plan

GRADE/AGE LEVEL: Ninth grade students

LESSON CONTENT: The Write Way Guidance Curriculum, in accordance with the Health/CSI curriculum, focuses on high school graduation readiness and requirements, college readiness information, and high school transition skills.

ASCA DOMAIN: Domain III: Personal/Social Development

Standard A: Students will acquire the attitudes, knowledge, and interpersonal skills to help them understand and respect self and others.

Competency 1: Acquire Self-Knowledge

Indicators:

a. develop positive attitudes toward self as a unique and worthy person;
b. identify values, attitudes, and beliefs;
c. learn the goal setting process;
d. understand change as a part of growth;
e. identify and express feelings;
f. distinguish between appropriate and inappropriate behavior;
g. recognize personal boundaries, rights, and privacy needs;
h. understand the need for self-control and how to practice it;
i. demonstrate proper behavior in groups;
j. identify personal strengths and assets.

CURRICULUM: Write Way Guidance Curriculum

START AND END DATES: October 2010 though May 2011

NUMBER OF STUDENTS AFFECTED: Approximately 436 students

LOCATION (where lesson is to be taught): Ninth Grade Health/CSI classrooms

EVALUATION AND ASSESSMENT: Pre and post student goal questionnaires, quarterly grades, quarterly referral reports, Write Way Curriculum Questionnaire

CONTACT PERSON: Molly Griffin *counselor.mgriffin@happymail.com* Gizelle Roberson *gizelle.roberson@happymail.com*

Appendix K: Guidance Curriculum Lesson Plan

GRADE/AGE LEVEL: Ninth grade students

LESSON CONTENT: The Write Way Guidance Curriculum, in accordance with the Health/CSI curriculum, focuses on high school graduation readiness and requirements, college readiness information, and high school transition skills.

ASCA DOMAIN: Domain III: Personal/Social Development

Standard A: Students will acquire the attitudes, knowledge, and interpersonal skills to help them understand and respect self and others.

Competency 1: Acquire Self-Knowledge

Indicators:

a. develop positive attitudes toward self as a unique and worthy person;
b. identify values, attitudes, and beliefs;
c. learn the goal setting process;
d. understand change as a part of growth;
e. identify and express feelings;
f. distinguish between appropriate and inappropriate behavior;
g. recognize personal boundaries, rights, and privacy needs;
h. understand the need for self-control and how to practice it;
i. demonstrate proper behavior in groups;
j. identify personal strengths and assets.

CURRICULUM: Write Way Guidance Curriculum

START AND END DATES: October 2010 though May 2011

NUMBER OF STUDENTS AFFECTED: Approximately 436 students

LESSON PLAN OVERVIEW:

Lesson One: Career Exploration Workshop (October 2010)
Career Cruising Activity

Lesson Two: The Story of School (November 2010)
This lesson is more of a personal/social activity involving the student reflecting on past successes and difficulties academically as well as problem solving and letter writing to an influential teacher.

Lesson Three: Graduation and College Requirements (December 2010)
This lesson includes reviewing graduation requirements and the A-G college requirements. Understanding credits.

Lesson Four: Four-Year Plans (January 2011)
This lesson is when we will be meeting during your W/Th block periods to meet individually with students to develop four-year plans.

Lesson Five: Understanding the Roles I Play (February 2011)
This lesson includes understanding roles that students can play in many areas of their life. They will identify when they are being participatory leaders and when they are being detractors in different situations.

Lesson Six: Problem Solving (March 2011)
Establishing problem solving skills as well as recognizing how each student solves their own problems. Discusses positive and negative outcomes as well as choice making and decision making skills.

Lesson Seven: Goals (April 2011)
Looking at where each student is and where they want to be. This brings in four-year plans, graduation and college requirements, roles students play in their lives, and skills to solve problems and reach goals.

Lesson Eight: Going For It! (May 2011)
In this final session, we will be having the students make collages and decorate their individual Write Way folders. They will also continue to reflect on their goals and will write a letter to themselves that we are hoping can be distributed either at the end of the 2010–2011 school year or at the beginning of the 2011–2012 school year.

Appendix K: Guidance Curriculum Results Report

GRADE/AGE LEVEL: Ninth grade students

LESSON CONTENT: The Write Way Guidance Curriculum, in accordance with the Health/CSI curriculum, focuses on high school graduation readiness and requirements, college readiness information, and high school transition skills.

ASCA DOMAIN: Domain III: Personal/Social Development

Standard A: Students will acquire the attitudes, knowledge, and interpersonal skills to help them understand and respect self and others.

Competency 1: Acquire Self-Knowledge

Indicators:

a. develop positive attitudes toward self as a unique and worthy person;
b. identify values, attitudes, and beliefs;

c. learn the goal setting process;
d. understand change as a part of growth;
e. identify and express feelings;
f. distinguish between appropriate and inappropriate behavior;
g. recognize personal boundaries, rights, and privacy needs;
h. understand the need for self-control and how to practice it;
i. demonstrate proper behavior in groups;
j. identify personal strengths and assets.

CURRICULUM: Write Way Guidance Curriculum

START AND END DATES: October 2010 though May 2011

NUMBER OF STUDENTS AFFECTED: Approximately 436 students

Appendix K: Assessment Instrument: Write Way Curriculum Questionnaire

Name: _____

Date: _____

In high school my goal is to: (*Circle one*)

JUST GET BY   ACHIEVE EXCELLENCE
1   2   3   4   5   6   7   8   9   10

What do you want to do after high school? *(Circle one)*

College   Work   Military   Other: _____

I have achieved _____ goal(s) I have set for myself. *(Circle one)*

0   1   2   3   4   5+

Someone who can help me achieve my goal is:

_____

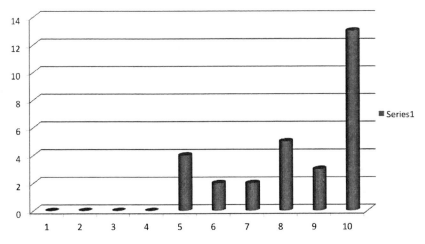

Figure K.2 In high school, my goal is to: _____

Appendix L
High School to Community College

Workshop Descriptions

- Session One: Introduction to the Community College System
- Session Two: Career and Major Exploration
- Session Three: The Community College Process
- Session Four: Completing the Application
- Session Five: The Importance of Financial Aid
- Session Six: The Importance of Placement Tests
- Session Seven: Special Programs and Resources
- Session Eight: Final Steps

Counseling Standards Addressed

- ACA Advocacy Standards
- ACA Multicultural Standards

Workshop Descriptions

Session One: Introduction to the Community College System

The introductory session focused on the benefits of attending community college and the various different pathways available through the community college system. At the end of the first session, there was a panel of speakers who shared their personal experiences of going through the community college system and transferring to a four-year university. Students completed the pre-program survey at the start of the session.

Session Two: Career and Major Exploration

To help students enter into community college with a more clear sense of what possible majors and careers they might be interested in, the second session focused on career and major exploration. Students completed an online career interest profile assessment through the California Colleges website and had the opportunity to research several possible careers of interest. At the end of the session, students examined the degree and certificate programs offered at SFBC and selected their top three to four programs of interest.

Session Three: The Community College Process

The third session built upon the background information from session one. In this session, students learned about the advantages of attending a community college, the cost, the transfer process, the benefits of meeting with a counselor to create a Student Education Plan, and an overview of the matriculation process at SFBC.

Session Four: Completing the Application

The fourth session was an open lab after school where students completed the online college application with the guidance of the school counselors.

Session Five: The Importance of Financial Aid

The fifth session was an informational session about financial aid for students and parents, followed by an open lab to complete the FAFSA or California Dream Act Application with the guidance of the school counselors.

Session Six: The Importance of Placement Tests

The sixth session provided students with background about the English and Math placement tests they are required to take as part of the matriculation process. We reviewed the importance of the assessments and showed students the Math and English course sequences, so they could see how placement would affect how long it would take to graduate/transfer. Students were given review materials to study and counselors reviewed the process of registering for the assessments.

Session Seven: Special Programs and Resources

The seventh session provided information on special programs and resources available to students at SFBC such as the Puente Project, Aspire, EOPS, MESA, and DSPS. Counselors reviewed the benefits of participation in special programs, qualification criteria, and the application process. The session concluded with a presentation by several alumni who were currently enrolled in special programs at SFBC. Students were given program applications at the end of the session.

Session Eight: Final Steps

In the eighth and final session, counselors reviewed the final steps in the matriculation and financial aid processes with students. Students completed the post-program survey. There was open lab time to help students complete any remaining final steps, such as reviewing assessment scores, completing the online orientation or registering for classes.

Counseling Standards Addressed

ACA Advocacy Standards

This research study addresses the following American Counseling Association's Advocacy Standards.

On behalf of the student, the counselor is able to:

- negotiate relevant services and educational systems;
- help students gain access to resources;
- develop a plan of action for confronting barriers;
- identify key allies in confronting those barriers.

In exerting systems change leadership at the school level, the counselor is able to:

- identify factors getting in the way of student success;
- collaborate with others to develop a plan for change;
- develop a step-by-step plan for implementing change.

ACA Multicultural Standards:

- Counselor awareness of own cultural background, beliefs and biases
- Counselor awareness of student's worldview and experiences
- Culturally appropriate intervention strategies

Bibliography

Adelman, C. (1993). Kurt Lewin and the origins of action research. *Educational Action Research*, 1(1), 7–24.

Adelman, H. S., & Taylor, L. (2006a). *The implementation guide to student learning supports in the classroom and schoolwide*. Thousand Oaks, CA: Corwin Press.

Adelman, H. S., & Taylor, L. (2006b). *The school leader's guide to student learning supports: New directions for addressing barriers to learning*. Thousand Oaks, CA: Corwin Press.

Ainsworth, P. K. (2010). *Developing a self-evaluating school: A practical guide*. London, UK: Continuum International Publishing.

Alexander, B. K. (2008). *The globalization of addiction: A study in poverty of the spirit*. Oxford, UK: Oxford University Press.

Alexander, B. K., & Shelton, C. P. (2014). *A history of psychology in western civilization*. Cambridge, UK: Cambridge University Press.

Alinsky, S. D. (1971). *Rules for radicals: A practical primer for realistic radicals*. New York: Vintage Books.

American School Counselor Association (ASCA). (2010). *Ethical standards for school counselors*. Alexandria, VA: Author.

American School Counselor Association (ASCA). (2012). *The ASCA national model: A framework for school counseling programs* (3rd ed.). Alexandria, VA: Author.

American School Counselor Association (ASCA). (2014). *Mindsets and behaviors for student success: K-12 college- and career-readiness standards for every student*. Alexandria, VA: Author.

Anthony, C. (1995). Ecopsychology and the deconstruction of whiteness. In T. Roszak, M. Gomes, & A. Kanner (Eds.), *Ecopsychology* (pp. 263–278). San Francisco, CA: Sierra Club Books.

Appiah, K. A. (2005). *The ethics of identity*. Princeton, NJ: Princeton University Press.

Archambault, R. D. (Ed.). (1964). *John Dewey on education: Selected writings*. Chicago, IL: University of Chicago Press.

Atkinson, T., & Claxton, G. (2000). *The intuitive practitioner: On the value of not always knowing what one is doing*. Philadelphia, PA: Open University Press.

Au, W., & Hollar, J. (2016, March 15). Opting out of the education reform industry. Retrieved from: https://rethinkingschoolsblog.wordpress.com/author/rethinkingschoolsblog/

Barrett, F. J. (2015). *Yes to the mess: Surprising leadership lessons from jazz*. Boston, MA: Harvard Business Review Press.

Barrett, F. J., & Fry, R. E. (2005). *Appreciative inquiry: A positive approach to building cooperative capacity*. Chagrin Falls, OH: Taos Institute Publications.

Beaudoin, M., & Taylor, M. (2004). *Creating a positive school culture: How principals and teachers can solve problems together*. Thousand Oaks, CA: Corwin Press.

Bemak, F., & Chung, R. (2005). Advocacy as a critical role for urban school counselors: Working toward equity and social justice. *Professional School Counseling, 8*(3), 196–202.

Benard, B. (1997). Changing the condition, place, and view of young people in society: An interview with youth development pioneer Bill Lofquist. *Resiliency in Action, 2*(1), 7–18.

Benard, B. (2004). *Resiliency: What we have learned*. San Francisco, CA: WestEd.

Benard, B., & Marshall, K. (1997). *A framework for practice: Tapping innate resiliency*. Minneapolis, MN: University of Minnesota, Center for Applied Research and Educational Improvement, College of Education and Human Development. Retrieved from: www.cehd.umn.edu/CAREI/Reports/Rpractice/Spring97/framework.html

Benard, B., & Slade, S. (2009). Listening to students: Moving resilience research to youth development practice and school connectedness. In R. Gilman, E. S. Huebner, & M. J. Furlong (Eds.), *Handbook of positive psychology in schools* (pp. 353–369). New York: Routledge.

Bender, F. L. (2003). *The culture of extinction: Toward a philosophy of deep ecology*. Amherst, NY: Humanity Books.

Bernstein, P. L. (1998). *Against the gods: The remarkable story of risk*. New York: John Wiley & Sons.

Bishop, M., & Vargas, C. (May 22, 2015). The invention of Hispanics. Latinousa. Retrieved from: http://latinousa.org/2015/05/22/the-invention-of-hispanics/

Bohm, D. (1996). *On dialogue*. New York: Routledge.

Bowers, C. A. (1997). *The culture of denial: Why the environmental movement needs a strategy for reforming universities and public school*. Albany, NY: State University of New York Press.

Bowers, C. A. (2000). *Let them eat data: How computers affect education, cultural diversity, and the prospects of ecological sustainability*. Athens, GA: The University of Georgia Press.

Bowers, C. A. (2001). *Educating for eco-justice and community*. Athens, GA: The University of Georgia Press.

Bowers, C. A. (2003). *Mindful conservatism: Rethinking the ideological and educational basis of an ecologically sustainable future*. Lanham, MD: Rowman & Littlefield.

Boyd, B. (2009). *On the origin of stories: Evolution, cognition, and fiction*. Cambridge, MA: Belknap Press.

Braidotti, R. (2013). *The posthuman*. Malden, MA: Polity Press.

Briscoe, F., Arriaza, G., & Henze, R. C. (2009). *The power of talk: How words change our lives*. Thousand Oaks, CA: Corwin.

Britton, J. (1970). *Language and learning*. New York: Penguin Books.

Bronfenbrenner, U. (1979). *The ecology of human development: Experiments by nature and design*. Cambridge, MA: Harvard University Press.

Brooks, R. B., & Goldstein, S. (2001). *Raising resilient children.* Lincolnwood, IL: Contemporary Books.

Bruner, J. S. (1986). *Actual minds, possible worlds.* Cambridge, MA: Harvard University Press.

Bruner, J. S. (1990). *Acts of meaning.* Cambridge, MA: Harvard University Press.

Bruner, J. S. (1996). *The culture of education.* Cambridge, MA: Harvard University Press.

Bruner, J. S. (2002). *Making stories: Law, literature, life.* New York: Farrar, Straus, & Giroux.

Brydon-Miller, M. (2008). Ethics and action research: Deepening our commitment to principles of social justice and redefining systems of democratic practice. In P. Reason & H. Bradbury (Eds.), *The Sage handbook of action research: Participative inquiry and practice* (2nd ed.) (pp. 199–210). Thousand Oaks, CA: Sage.

Bryk, A., Sebring, P., Allensworth, E., Luppesco, S., & Easton, J. (2010). *Organizing schools for improvement: Lessons from Chicago.* Chicago, IL: University of Chicago Press.

Buber, M. (1970). *I and Thou.* New York: Charles Scribner's Sons.

Burns, G. W. (1998). *Nature-guided therapy: Brief integrative strategies for health and well-being.* Philadelphia, PA: Brunner/Mazel.

Burr, V. (1995). *An introduction to social constructionism.* London: Routledge.

Buzzell, L., & Chalquist, C. (Eds.). (2009). *Ecotherapy: Healing with nature in mind.* San Francisco, CA: Sierra Club Books.

Cahill, C. (2007). Doing research with young people: Participatory research and the rituals of collective work. *Children's Geographies, 5*(3), 297–312.

California Department of Education. (2007). *California results-based school counseling and student support guidelines.* Sacramento, CA: Author.

Capra, F. (1996). *The web of life: A new scientific understanding of living systems.* New York: Anchor Books.

Capra, F. (2002). *The hidden connections: Integrating the biological, cognitive, and social dimensions of life into a science of sustainability.* New York: Random House.

Caputo, J. D. (1993). *Against ethics: Contributions to a poetics of obligation with constant reference to deconstruction.* Bloomington, IN: Indiana University Press.

Chappuis, J. (2009). *Seven strategies of assessment for learning.* Portland, OR: Educational Testing Service.

Chappuis, S., Stiggins, R. J., Arter, J., & Chappuis, J. (2005). *Assessment for learning: An action guide for school leaders.* Portland, OR: Educational Testing Service.

Chevalier, J. M., & Buckles, D. J. (2013) *Handbook for participatory action research, planning and evaluation.* Ottawa: SAS2 Dialogue.

Claxton, G. (1997). *Hare brain, tortoise mind: Why intelligence increases when you think less.* Hopewell, NJ: Ecco Press.

Claxton, G. (1999). *Wise up: The challenge of lifelong learning.* New York: Bloomsbury.

Claxton, G. (2002). *Building learning power: Helping young people become better learners.* Bristol, UK: TLO.

Claxton, G. (2008). *What's the point of school?: Rediscovering the heart of education.* Oxford, UK: Oneworld Publications.

230   *Bibliography*

Claxton, G., & Lucas, B. (2015). *Educating Ruby: What our children really need to learn.* Cafmarthen, Wales, UK: Crown House Publishing.

Claxton, G., Chambers, M., Powell, G., & Lucas, B. (2011). *The learning powered school: Pioneering 21st century education.* Bristol, UK: TLO.

CollegeMeasures.org. *CollegeMeasures.org—2-Year College Data Tool.* Retrieved March 8, 2014 from: http://collegemeasures.org/2-year_colleges/home/

Comstock, D. (2005). *Diversity and development: Critical contexts that share our lives and relationships.* Belmont, CA: Thomson Brooks/Cole.

Comstock, D. L., Hammer, T. R., Strentzsch, J., Cannon, K., Parsons, J., & Salazar, G. (2008). Relational–cultural theory: A framework for bridging relational, multicultural, and social justice competencies. *Journal of Counseling and Development*, 86(3), 279–287.

Conyne, R. K., & Cook, E. P. (Eds.). (2004). *Ecological counseling: An innovative approach to conceptualizing person-environment interaction.* Alexandria, VA: American Counseling Association.

Cooperrider, D. L., & Whitney, D. (1999). *Appreciative inquiry: Collaborating for change.* San Francisco, CA: Barrett-Koehler.

Cooperrider, D. L., & Whitney, D. (2005). *Appreciative inquiry: A positive revolution in change.* San Francisco, CA: Barrett-Koehler.

Cooperrider, D. L., Whitney, D., & Stavros, J. M. (2003). *Appreciative inquiry handbook: The first in a series of AI workbooks for leaders of change.* Bedford, OH: Lakeshore Publishers.

Copland, M. A. (2003). Leadership of inquiry: Building and sustaining capacity for school improvement. *Educational Evaluation and Policy Analysis*, 25(4), 375–395.

Coyle, D. (2009). *The talent code: Greatness isn't born. It's grown. Here's how.* New York: Bantam.

Crosnoe, R., Johnson, M. K., & Elder Jr., G. H. (2004). Intergenerational bonding in school: The behavioral and contextual correlates of student-teacher relationships. *Sociology in Education*, 77(1), 60–81.

Csikszentmihalyi, M. (1990). *Flow: The psychology of optimal experience.* New York: Harper & Row.

Csikszentmihalyi, M., Rathunde, K., Whalen, S., & Wong, M. (1993). *Talented teenagers: The roots of success and failure.* New York: Cambridge University Press.

Cummings, J. (1986). Empowering minority students: A framework for intervention. *Harvard Education Review*, 56(1), 18–36.

Cupitt, D. (1995). *Solar ethics.* London: SCM Press.

Cupitt, D. (1999). *The new religion of life in everyday speech.* London: SCM Press.

Cupitt, D. (2003). *Life, life.* Santa Rosa, CA: Polebridge Press.

Dana, N. F. (2013). *Digging deeper into action research: A teacher inquirer's field guide.* Thousand Oaks, CA: Corwin.

Darling-Hammond, L., Chung Wei, R., Andree, A., Richardson, N., & Orphanos, S. (2009). *Professional learning in the learning profession: A status report on teacher development in the United States and abroad.* Dallas, TX: National Staff Development Council.

Davis, J., & Martin, D. (2008). Racism, assessment, and instructional practices: Implications for mathematics teachers of African American students. *Journal of Urban Mathematics Education*, 1(10), 10–34.

Davis, W. (2007). *Light at the edge of the world: A journey through the realm of vanishing cultures.* Vancouver, BC: Douglas & McIntyre.

Delpit, L. (1995). *Other people's children: Cultural conflict in the classroom.* New York: The New Press.

Delpit, L. (2006). Lessons from teachers. *Journal of Teacher Education, 57*(3), 220–231.

Dewey, J. (1929/1960). *The quest for certainty: A study of the relation of knowledge and action.* New York: Capricorn Books.

Dewey, J. (1938). *Education and experience.* New York: Collier Books.

Diamond, J. (1999). *Guns, germs, and steel: The fates of human societies.* New York: W. W. Norton.

Dimmitt, C., Carey, J. C., & Hatch, T. (2007). *Evidence-based school counseling: Making a difference with data-driven practices.* Thousand Oaks, CA: Corwin Press.

Dole, D., Godwin, L., & Moehle, M. (Story Curators) (2014). *Exceeding expectations: An anthology of appreciative inquiry stories in education from around the world.* Chagrin Falls, OH: Taos Institute. Publications/WorldShare Books and the authors of each story.

Dowdy, E., Furlong, M., Raines, T. C., Bovery, B., Kauffman, B., Kamphaus, R. W., Dever, B. V., Price, M., & Murdock, J. (2015). Enhancing school-based mental health services with a preventive and promotive approach to universal screening for complete mental health. *Journal of Educational and Psychological Consultation, 25,* 1–20.

Dragonas, T., Gergen, K., McNamee, S., & Tseliou, E. (Eds.). (2015). *Education as social construction: Contributions to theory, research, and practice.* Chagrin Falls, OH: Taos Books Publications/WorldShare Books.

DuFour, R. (2006). *Learning by doing: a handbook for professional learning communities at work.* Bloomington, IN: Solution Tree.

Dweck, C. S. (2006). *Mindset: The new psychology of success.* New York: Random House.

Education Trust. (2000). *National initiative for transforming school counseling summer academy for counselor educators proceedings.* Washington, DC: Author.

Efran, J. S., Lukens, M. D., & Lukens, R. J. (1990). *Language, structure, and change: Frameworks for meaning in psychotherapy.* New York: Norton.

Einstein, A. (1950). Letters of Note, Einstein letter to Robert S. Marcus, http://www.lettersofnote.com/2011/11/delusion.html

Ellis, D., & Hughes, K. (2002). *Partnerships by design: Cultivating effective and meaningful school–family–community partnerships.* Portland, OR: Northwest Regional Educational Laboratory.

Field, J. E., & Baker, S. (2004). Defining and examining school counselor advocacy. *Professional School Counseling, 8*(1), 56–63.

Finser, T. M. (2007). *Silence is complicity: A call to let teachers improve our schools through action research—not NCLB.* Great Barrington, MA: Steiner Books.

Fletcher, J. (1966). *Situation ethics: A new morality.* Philadelphia, PA: The Westminster Press.

Freire, P. (1997). *The pedagogy of hope: Reliving the pedagogy of the oppressed.* New York: Continuum Publishing.

Fullan, M. (2001). *Leading in a culture of change.* San Francisco, CA: Jossey-Bass.

Furlong, M. J., You, S., Renshaw, T. L., Smith, D. C., & O'Malley, M. D. (2013). Preliminary development and validation of the Social and Emotional Health Survey for secondary students. *Social Indicators Research*. First published online June 27, 2103. Retrieved July 28, 2016 from: http://search.proquest.com. proxylib.csueastbay.edu/docview/1531573887?accountid=28458

Galassi, J. P., & Akos, P. (2007). *Strengths-based school counseling: Promoting student development and achievement*. Mahwah, NJ: Lawrence Erlbaum Associates.

Gandara, P., Alvarado, E., Driscoll, A., & Orfield, G. (2012). Building pathways to transfer: Community colleges that break the chain of failure for students of color. *UCLA Civil Rights Project*, 1–117. Retrieved from: http://files.eric.ed.gov/fulltext/ED529493.pdf

Gandhi, M. K. (1953). *Towards new education*. Ahmedabad, India: Navjivan Press.

Gergen, K. J. (2006). *Therapeutic realities: Collaboration, oppression and relational flow*. Chagrin Falls, OH: Taos Institute Publications.

Gergen, K. J. (2009). *Relational being: Beyond self and community*. New York: Oxford University Press.

Gergen, K. J. (2015). From mirroring to world-making: Research as future forming. *Journal for the Theory of Social Behaviour*, 45(3), 287–310.

Gergen, K. J. & Gergen, M. M. (2008). Social construction and research as action. In P. Reason & H. Bradbury. *The Sage handbook of action research: Participative inquiry and practice* (2nd ed.). (pp. 159–171). Thousand Oaks, CA: Sage.

Gibbs, J. (2001). *Tribes: A new way of learning and being together*. Windsor, CA: Center Source.

Gibbs, J. (2006). *Reaching all by creating tribes learning communities*. Windsor, CA: Center Source.

Gilbert, P. (2009). *The compassionate mind: A new approach to life's challenges*. Oakland, CA: New Harbinger Publications.

Gillen, J. (2014). *Educating for insurgency: The roles of young people in schools of poverty*. Oakland, CA: AK Press.

Global Warming Science. (n.d.). Retrieved March 21, 2016 from: www.ucsusa.org/our-work/global-warming/science-and-impacts/global-warming-science#. VvA_9mQrJWM

Goddard, Y. L., Goddard, R. D., & Tschannen-Moran, M. (2007). A theoretical and empirical investigation of teacher collaboration for school improvement and student achievement in public elementary schools. *Teachers College Record*, 109(4), 877–896.

Goldberg, E. (2001). *The executive brain: Frontal lobes and the civilized mind*. New York: Oxford University Press.

Goleman, D. (2013). *Focus: The hidden driver of excellence*. New York, NY: HarperCollins.

Goleman, D. (2015). *A force for good: The Dalai Lama's vision for our world*. London, UK: Bloomsbury.

Goleman, D., Bennett, L., & Barlow, Z. (2012). *Ecoliterate: How educators are cultivating emotional, social, and ecological intelligence*. San Francisco, CA: Jossey-Bass Publishers.

Goodlad, J. I., & McMannon, T. J. (1997). *The public purpose of education and schooling*. San Francisco, CA: Jossey-Bass Publishers.

Goodman, P. (1960). *Growing up absurd: Problems of youth in the organized society.* New York: Vintage Books.

Gottschall, J. (2012). *The storytelling animal: How stories make us human.* New York: Houghton Mifflin Harcourt.

Greason, P. B., & Cashwell, C. S. (2009). Mindfulness and counseling self-efficacy: The mediating role of attention and empathy. *Counselor Education and Supervision, 49*(1), 2–19.

Griffin, D., & Farris, A. (2010). School counselors and collaboration: Finding resources through community asset mapping. *Professional School Counseling, 13*(5), 248–256.

Guskey, T. (2000). *Evaluating professional development.* Thousand Oaks, CA: Corwin.

Gysbers, N. C, & Henderson, P. (2012). *Developing and managing your school guidance and counseling program* (5th ed.). Alexandria, VA: American Counseling Association.

Hagopian, J. (2016, March 19). Six reasons why the revolt against standardized testing is good for students and parents of color. Retrieved from: https://moveto amend.org/six-reasons-why-revolt-against-standardized-testing-good-students-and-parents-color

Haidt, J. (2006). *The happiness hypothesis: Finding modern truth in ancient wisdom.* New York: Basic Books.

Haidt, J. (2012). *The righteous mind: Why good people are divided by politics and religion.* New York: Pantheon Books.

Hansen, J. T. (2004). Thoughts on knowing: Epistemic implications of counseling practice. *Journal of Counseling & Development, 82,* 131–138.

Hansen, J. T. (2005a). Postmodernism and humanism: A proposed integration of perspectives that value human meaning systems. *Journal of Humanistic Counseling Education and Development, 44*(1), 3–15.

Hansen, J. T. (2005b). The devaluation of inner subjective experiences by the counseling profession: A plea to reclaim the essence of the profession. *Journal of Counseling & Development, 83*(4), 406–415.

Hansen, J. T. (2006a). Humanism as moral imperative: Comments on the role of knowing in the helping encounter. *Journal of Humanistic Counseling, Education and Development, 45*(2), 115–125.

Hansen, J. T. (2006b). Counseling theories within a postmodernist epistemology: New roles for theories in counseling practice. *Journal of Counseling & Development, 84*(3), 291–297.

Hansen, J. T. (2007). Counseling without truth: Toward a neopragmatic foundation for counseling practice. *Journal of Counseling and Development, 85,* 423–430.

Hansen, J. (2009). On displaced humanists: Counselor education and the meaning-reduction pendulum. *Journal of Humanistic Counseling, Education and Development, 48*(1), 65–76.

Hanson, T. L., Austin, G., & Lee-Bayha, J. (2004*). Ensuring that no child is left behind: How are student health risks and resilience related to the academic progress of schools?* San Francisco, CA: WestEd.

Harris, J., Davidson, L., Hayes, B., Humphreys, K., LaMarca, P., Berliner, B., Poynor, L., & Van Houten, L. (2014). *Speak out, listen up! Tools for using student perspectives and local data for school improvement* (REL 2014–035). Washington, DC: U.S. Department of Education, Institute of Education Sciences,

National Center for Education Evaluation and Regional Assistance, Regional Educational Laboratory West. Retrieved from: http://ies. ed.gov/ncee/edlabs

Hatch, T. (2007). Using the flashlight builder approach to measuring and sharing results! The Center for Excellence in School Counseling and Leadership (CESCaL). Retrieved from: www.cescal.org/flashlight.cfm.

Hatch, T. (2014). *The use of data in school counseling: Hatching results for students, programs and the profession.* Thousand Oaks, CA: Corwin.

Hatch, T., & Lewis, R. E. (2011). *Promoting social justice with wisdom and data.* Retrieved from: http://counselingoutfitters.com/vistas/vistas11/Article_xx.pdf

Hayes, S. C., Hayes, L. J., Reese, H. W., & Sarbin, T. R. (Eds.). (1993). *Varieties of scientific contextualism.* Reno, NV: Context Press.

Health and Human Development Program (2011). *Workbook for improving school climate.* Los Alamitos: WestEd. Available for download at californias3. wested.org

Herman, J. L., & Gribbons, B. (2001). Lessons learned in using data to support school inquiry and continuous improvement: Final report to the Stuart Foundation (CSE Technical Report No. 535). Los Angeles, CA: Center for the Study of Evaluation, University of California, Los Angeles.

Heron, J., & Reason, P. (1997). A participatory inquiry paradigm. *Qualitative Inquiry, 3,* 274–294.

Herr, K., & Anderson, G. L. (2005). *The action research dissertation: A guide for students and faculty.* Thousand Oaks, CA: Sage.

Holcomb-McCoy, C. (2007). *School counseling to close the achievement gap: A social justice framework for success.* Thousand Oaks, CA: Corwin Press.

Holzman, L. (1997). *Schools for growth: Radical alternatives to current educational models.* Mahwah, NJ: Lawrence Erlbaum.

House, R. M., & Martin, P. J. (1998). Advocating for better futures for all students: A new vision for school counselors. *Education, 119,* 284–291.

Huffman, D., & Kalnin, J. (2003). Collaborative inquiry to make data-based decisions in schools. *Teaching and Teacher Education, 19,* 569–580.

Hunt, J. (2003). *No dream denied: A pledge to America's children.* Washington, DC: National Commission on Teaching and America's Future.

Hunt, J., & Carrol, T. G. (2003). *No dream denied: A pledge to America's children.* Washington, DC: Summary Report of National Commission on Teaching and America's Future.

Husserl, E. (1970; originally published 1936). *The crisis of European sciences and transcendental phenomenology: An introduction to phenomenological philosophy.* Evanston, IL: Northwestern University Press.

Ingold, T. (2011). *Being alive: Essays on movement, knowledge, and description.* New York, NY: Routledge.

Isaacs, W. (1999). *Dialogue and the art of thinking together.* New York: Currency Book.

Ivey, A., Ivey, M., Myers, J., & Sweeney, T. (2005). *Developmental counseling and therapy: Promoting wellness over the lifespan.* Boston, MA: Lahaska Press.

Ivey, A. E., Packard, N. G., & Ivey, M. B. (2006). *Basic attending skills* (4th ed.). Framingham, MA: Microtraining Associates.

Jackson, L. D. (2009). Revisiting adult learning theory through the lens of an adult learner. *Adult Learning, 20*(3–4), 20–22.

James, W. (1912/2003). *Essays in radical empiricism.* Mineola, NY: Dover Publications.

Jennings, G. (2012). Finding professional mojo in schools: Authentic motivation, satisfaction, and identity. Unpublished paper presented May 22, 2012, California State University, East Bay, Hayward, CA.

Jennings, G., & Tran, O. K. (2009, February). The impact of asset gaps: Implications for service and training. Poster presentation presented at the National Association of School Psychologists, Boston, MA.

Jia, Y., Way, N., Ling, G., Yoshikawa, H., Chen, X., Hughes, D., Ke, X., & Lu, Z. (2009). The influence of student perceptions of school climate on socio-emotional and academic adjustment: A comparison of Chinese and American adolescents. *Child Development, 80*(5), 1514–1530.

Johnson, S., Johnson, C., & Downs, L. (2006). *Building a results-based student support program.* Boston, MA: Lahaska Press.

Kabat-Zinn, J. (1994). *Wherever you go, there you are.* New York: Hyperion.

Kahneman, D. (2011). *Thinking, fast and slow.* New York: Farrar, Straus, and Giroux.

Kapyrka, J., & Dockstator, M. (2012). Indigenous knowledges and Western knowledges in environmental education: Acknowledging the tensions for the benefits of a "two-worlds" approach. *Canadian Journal of Environmental Education, 17,* 97–112.

Karcher, M., & Sass, D. (2010). A multicultural assessment of adolescent connectedness: Testing measurement invariance across gender and ethnicity. *Journal of Counseling Psychology, 57*(3), 274–289.

Kasser, T., & Kanner, A. D. (Eds.). (2004). *Psychology and consumer culture: The struggle for a good life in a materialistic world.* Washington, DC: American Psychological Association.

Kearney, R. (2002). *On stories.* New York: Routledge.

Kelly, J. G. (2000). Wellness as an ecological enterprise. In D. Cicchetti, J. Rappaport, I. Sandler, & R. P. Weissberg (Eds.), *The promotion of wellness in children and adolescents* (pp. 101–131). Washington, DC: CWLA Press.

Keltner, D. (2009). *Born to be good: The science of a meaningful life.* New York: W. W. Norton.

Krueger, R. A., & Casey, M. A. (2009). *Focus groups: A practical guide for applied research* (4th ed.). Thousand Oaks, CA: Sage Publications.

Lakoff, G., & Johnson, M. (1999). *Philosophy in the flesh: The embodied mind and its challenge to Western thought.* New York: Basic Books.

Lambert, L. (2003). Leadership redefined: An evocative context for teacher leadership. *School Leadership and Management, 23*(4), 423–430.

Langer, E. J. (1989). *Mindfulness.* Reading, MA: Addison-Wesley.

Larson, K. N, Grudens-Schuck, N., & Lundy Allen, B. (2004). Can you call it a focus group? Ames, IO: Iowa State Extension. Retrieved from: www.extension.iastate.edu/Publications/PM1969A.pdf

Lawson, H. (2001). *Closure: A story of everything.* New York: Routledge.

Lee, C. C. (Ed.). (2007). *Counseling for social justice* (2nd ed.). Alexandria, VA: American Counseling Association.

Leopold, A. (1949). *A sand county almanac and sketches here and there.* New York: Oxford University Press.

Lewin, K. (1936). *Principles of topological psychology.* New York, NY: McGraw-Hill.

Lewis, C., Perry, R., Hurd, J., & O'Connell, M. P. (2006). Lesson study comes of age in North America. *Phi Delta Kappan, 88*(4), 273–281.

Lewis, J. A., Arnold, M. S., House, R., & Toporek, R. L. (2002). *Advocacy competencies: Task force on advocacy competencies.* Alexandria, VA: American Counseling Association.

Lewis, R. E. (1999) A write way: Fostering resiliency during transitions. *Journal of Humanistic Education and Development, 37*, 200–211.

Lewis, R. E. (2000). Hope in the new millennium. *The Counselor: A Publication of the Oregon Counseling Association, 11*(5), 1–2.

Lewis, R. E. (2007). Resilience in individuals, families, and communities. In D. Capuzzi and D. R. Gross (Eds.), *Youth at risk* (5th ed.) (pp. 39–68). Alexandria, VA: American Counseling Association.

Lewis, R. E. (2010). An ecological model. *Educational Psychology.* California State University, East Bay.

Lewis, R. E. (2011). Ecohumanism: Integrating humanism with resilience theory. In M. B. Scholl, A. S. McGowan, & J. T. Hansen (Eds.), *Humanistic perspectives on contemporary counseling issues* (pp. 191–214). New York, NY: Routledge.

Lewis, R. E. (2013). What color is your heart? Personalizing humanism. In R. M. Borunda, *What color is your heart?: A humanist approach to diversity* (2nd ed.) (pp. 167–184). Dubuque, IA: Kendall Hunt.

Lewis, R. E. (2014). Resilience in individuals, families, and communities. In D. Capuzzi & D. R. Gross (Eds.), *Youth at risk* (6th ed.) (pp. 43–65). Alexandria, VA: American Counseling Association.

Lewis, R. E., & Borunda, R. (2006). Lived stories: Participatory leadership in action. *Journal of Counseling and Development, 84*, 406–413.

Lewis, R. E., & Emil, S. (2010). Appreciative inquiry: A pilot study of school counselor graduates. *Journal of Humanistic Counseling, Education and Development, 49*(1), 98–111.

Lewis, R. E., & Hatch, T. (2008). Cultivating strengths-based professional identities. *Professional School Counseling, 12*(2), 115–118.

Lewis, R. E., & Winkelman, P. (2014). Four phases and nine steps in the participatory inquiry process. *Educational Psychology.* California State University, East Bay.

Lewis, R. E., Lenski, S. D., Mukhopadhyay, S., & Cartwright, C. T. (2010). Mindful wonderment: Using focus groups to frame social justice. *Journal for Social Action in Counseling and Psychology, 2*, 82–105.

Lindsey, R. B., Lindsey, D. B., & Terrell, R. D. (2011). Focusing on assets to overcome barriers. In A. M. Blankstein, & P. D. Houston (Eds.), *Leadership for social justice and democracy in our schools* (pp. 25–43). Thousand Oaks, CA: Corwin.

Linell, P. (2009). *Rethinking language, mind, and world dialogically: Interactional and contextual theories of human sense-making.* Charlotte, NC: Information Age Publishing.

Liu, E., & Hanauer, N. (2011). *The gardens of democracy: A new American story of citizenship, the economy, and the role of government.* Seattle, WA: Sasquatch Books.

Loesch, L. C. (2007). Fair access to and use of assessment in counseling. In C. C. Lee (Ed.), *Counseling for social justice* (2nd ed.) (pp. 201–222). Alexandria, VA: American Counseling Association.

Louis, K. S. (1994). Beyond "managed change": Rethinking how schools improve. *School Effectiveness and School Improvement, 9*(1), 1–27.

Louis, K. S., & Marks, H. (1998). Does professional learning community affect the classroom? Teachers' work and student experience in restructured schools. *American Journal of Education, 106*(4), 532–575.

Ludema, J. D., Cooperrider, D. L., & Barrett, F. J. (2000). Appreciative inquiry: The power of the unconditional positive question. In P. Reason & H. Bradbury (Eds.), *Handbook of action research: Participative inquiry and practice* (pp. 189–199). London: Sage Publications.

McWhorter, J. (2001). *The power of Babel: A natural history of language.* New York: Perennial.

Macy, J., & Johnstone, C. (2012). *Active hope: How to face the mess we're in without going crazy.* Novato, CA: New World Library.

Masten, A. S. (2001). Ordinary magic: Resilience processes in development. *American Psychologist, 56,* 227–238.

Masten, A. S. (2007). Resilience in developing systems: Progress and promise as the fourth wave rises. *Development and Psychopathology, 19*(3), 921–930.

Masten, A. S. (2014). *Ordinary magic: Resilience in development.* New York: Guilford Press.

Masten, A. S., & Coatsworth, J. D. (1998). The development of competence in favorable and unfavorable environments. *American Psychologist, 53,* 205–220.

Masten, A. S., Herbers, J. E., Cutuli, J. J., & Lafavor, T. L. (2008). Promoting competence and resilience in the school context. *Professional School Counseling, 12*(2), 76–84.

Masten, A. S., Cutuli, J. J., Herbers, J. E., & Reed, M. J. (2009). Resilience in development. In S. J. Lopez & C. R. Snyder (Eds.), *Oxford handbook of positive psychology* (pp. 117–131). New York: Oxford University Press.

Mead, G. H. (1932/2002). *The philosophy of the present.* Amherst, NY: Prometheus Books.

Mead, G. H. (1934/1967). *Mind, self, and society from the standpoint of a social behaviorist.* Chicago, IL: University of Chicago Press.

Mehl-Madrona, L. (2005). *Coyote wisdom: The power of story in healing.* Rochester, VT: Bear and Company.

Mehl-Madrona, L. (2007). *Narrative medicine: The use of history and story in the healing process.* Rochester, VT: Bear and Company.

Mehl-Madrona, L. (2010). *Healing the mind through the power of story: The promise of narrative psychiatry.* Rochester, VT: Bear and Company.

Miller, B. D., & Duncan, B. L. (2000). *The outcome and session rating scales* [Administration and Scoring Manual]. Chicago, IL: Institute for the Study of Therapeutic Change.

Miller, J., & Garran, A. M. (2008). *Racism in the United States: Implications for the helping professions.* Belmont, CA: Brooks/Cole.

Milton, K. (2002). *Loving nature: Towards an ecology of emotion.* New York: Routledge.

Monk, G., Winslade, J., Crocket, K., & Epston, D. (Eds.). (1997). *Narrative therapy in practice: The archaeology of hope.* San Francisco, CA: Jossey-Bass.

Morin, E., & Kern, A. B. (1999). *Homeland earth.* Cresskill, NJ: Hampton Press.

Moses, R. P. (2001). *Radical equations: Math literacy and civil rights.* Boston, MA: Beacon Press.

Muir, J. (1894/1961). *The mountains of California.* Garden City, NY: The Natural History Library.

Myers, J. E., & Sweeney, T. J. (Eds.). (2005). *Counseling for wellness: Theory, research, and practice.* Alexandria, VA: American Counseling Association.

Naess, A. (1988). Self-realization: An ecological approach to being in the world. In J. Seed, J. Macy, P. Fleming, & A. Naess (Eds.), *Thinking like a mountain: Towards a council of all beings* (pp. 19–30). Santa Cruz, CA: New Society Publishers.

Naess, A. (2002). *Life's philosophy: reason and feeling in a deeper world.* Athens, GA: University of Georgia Press.

Nash, R. F. (1989). *The rights of nature: A history of environmental ethics.* Madison, WI: University of Wisconsin Press.

National Commission on Excellence in Education. (1983). *A nation at risk: The imperative for educational reform. A report to the nation and the Secretary of Education, United States Department of Education.* Washington, DC: Author.

Neufeldt, S. A., & Nelson, M. L. (2004). Ecological counselling: Constructionist and postmodern perspectives. In R. K. Conyne & E. P. Cook (Eds.), *Ecological counseling: An innovative approach to conceptualizing person-environment interaction.* Alexandria, VA: American Counselng Association.

Newbury, J. (2014). Inquiring into life as we live it. *Child and Youth Services, 35,* 196–215.

Newman, F., & Holzman, L. (1993). *Lev Vygotsky: Revolutionary scientist.* New York: Routledge.

Newman, F., & Holzman, L. (1996). *Unscientific psychology: A cultural-performatory approach to understanding human life.* Westport, CT: Praeger Publishers.

Noguera, P. A. (2003). *City schools and the American dream: Reclaiming the promise of public education.* New York: Teacher College Press.

Obrist, H. U. (2011). *Ai Weiwei speaks with Hans Urich Obrist.* London: Penguin Books.

Odden, A. R., & Archibald, S. (2009). *Doubling student performance . . . and finding the resources to do it.* San Francisco, CA: Corwin Press.

O'Malley, M. D., & Amarillas, A. (2011). *What works brief #1: Caring relationships and high expectations.* Los Alamitos, CA: WestEd. Available for download at: http://californias3.wested.org/tools/s

Paisley, P. O., & Hubbard, G. T. (1994). *Developmental school counseling programs: From theory to practice.* Alexandria, VA: American Counseling Association.

Peavy, R. V. (2004). *Sociodynamic counseling: A practical approach to meaning making.* Chagrin Falls, OH: Taos Institute.

Peirce, C. S. (1923/1998). *Chance, love, and logic: Philosophical essays.* Lincoln, NE: University of Nebraska Press.

Pepper, S. C. (1942). *World hypotheses: A study in evidence.* Berkeley, CA: University of California Press.

Preskill, H., & Catsambas, T. T. (2006). *Reframing evaluation through appreciative inquiry.* Thousand Oaks, CA: Sage.

Prilleltensky, I., & Prilleltensky, O. (2005). Beyond resilience: Blending wellness and liberation in the helping professions. In M. Ungar (Ed.), *Handbook for working with children and youth: Pathways to resilience across cultures and contexts* (pp. 89–103). Thousand Oaks, CA: Sage.

Prilleltensky, I., & Prilleltensky, O. (2006). *Promoting well-being: Linking personal, organizational, and community change.* Hoboken, NJ: John Wiley & Sons.

Prochaska, J., Norcross, J., & DiClemente, C. (1994). *Changing for good.* New York: Avon Books.

Puente Project. (2014). PUENTE'S 30th anniversary: Helping underserved students achieve for 30 years. *The Puente Project.* Retrieved March 8, 2014 from: www.puente.net/

Ratts, M. J., DeKruyf, L., & Chen-Hayes, S. F. (2007). The ACA advocacy competencies: A social justice advocacy framework for professional school counselors. *Professional School Counseling, 11,* 90–97.

Ravitch, D. (2016, March 24). Solving the mystery of the schools [Review of the books *The prize: Who's in charge of America's schools?, by D. Russakoff and Mission High: One school, how experts tried to fail it, and the students and teachers who made it triumph,* by K. Rizga]. *The New York Review of Books, 63*(5), 34–36.

Reason, P. & Bradbury, H. (2001*). Handbook of action research: Participative inquiry and practice.* Thousand Oaks, CA: Sage.

Reason, P., & Bradbury, H. (2008). *The Sage handbook of action research: Participative inquiry and practice* (2nd ed.). Thousand Oaks, CA: Sage.

Reason, P., & Hawkins, P. (1988). Story telling as inquiry. In P. Reason (Ed.), *Human inquiry in action: Developments in new paradigm research* (pp. 79–101). London: Sage.

Renshaw, T. L., Furlong, M. J., Dowdy, E., Rebelez, J., Smith, D. C., O'Malley, M., Lee, S. L., & Strom, I. F. (2014). Covitality: A synergistic conception of adolescents' mental health. In M. J. Furlong, R. Gilman, & E. S. Huebner (Eds.), *Handbook of positive psychology in the schools* (2nd ed.) (pp. 12–32). New York, NY: Routledge/Taylor & Francis.

Rowell, L. (2005). Collaborative action research and school counselors. *Professional School Counseling, 9*(1), 28–36.

Rowell, L. (2006). Action research and school counseling: Closing the gap between research and practice. *Professional School Counseling, 9*(5), 376–384.

School Accountability Report Card (SARC). (2009). Hayward High School. Hayward, CA: Hayward Unified School District. Retrieved from: http://hayward. schoolwisepress.com/home/site.aspx?entity=12267

Schor, J. B. (1998). *The overspent American: Why we want what we don't need.* New York: Basic Books.

Schumacher, E. F. (1973). *Small is beautiful: Economics as if people mattered.* New York: Harper Row.

Sessions, G. (Ed.). (1995). *Deep ecology for the 21st century: Readings on the philosophy and practice of the new environmentalism.* Boston, MA: Shambhala.

Sheldrake, P. (2014). *Spirituality: A guide for the perplexed.* New York, NY: Bloomsbury.

Siegel, D. J. (2010). *Mindsight: The new science of personal transformation.* New York: Bantam Books.

Siegel, D. J. (2012). *The developing mind: How relationships and the brain interact to shape who we are* (2nd ed.). New York: Guilford Press.

Skiba, R., Horner, R., Chung, C. G., Rausch, M. K., May, S., & Tobin, T. (2011). Race is not neutral: A national investigation of African American and Latino disproportionality in school discipline. *School Psychology Review, 40*(1), 85–107.

Skolimowski, H. (1993). *A sacred place to dwell: Living with reverence upon the earth.* Boston, MA: Element Books.

Skolimowski, H. (1994). *The participatory mind: A new theory of knowledge and of the universe.* London: Penguin.

Smith, F. (1975). *Comprehension and learning: A conceptual framework for teachers.* New York: Holt, Rinehart, & Winston.

Smith, F. (1982). *Writing and the writer.* New York: Holt, Rinehart, and Winston.

Smith, F. (1986). *Insult to intelligence: Bureaucratic invasion of our classrooms.* New York: Arbor House.

Smith, F. (1998). *The book of learning and forgetting.* New York: Teachers College Press.

Smith, F. (2006). *Ourselves: Why we are who we are; a handbook for educators.* Mahwah, NJ: Lawrence Erlbaum Associates.

Smith, G. A., & Williams, D. R. (Eds.). (1999). *Ecological education in action: On weaving education, culture, and the environment.* Albany, NY: State University of New York Press.

Sobel, D. (2004). *Place-based education: Connecting classrooms and communities.* Great Barrington, MA: Orion Society.

Solnit, R. (2006). *Hope in the dark: Untold histories, wild possibilities.* New York: Nation Books.

Solnit, R. (2014). *Men explain things to me.* Chicago, IL: Haymarket Books.

Somekh, B., & Zeichner, K. (2009). Action research for educational reform: Remodeling action research theories and practices in local contexts. *Educational Action Research, 17,* 5–21.

Spretnak, C. (2011). *Relational reality: New discoveries of interrelatedness that are transforming the modern world.* Topsham, ME: Green Horizons Books.

Squier, K. L., Nailor, P., & Carey, J. C. (2014). *Achieving excellence in school counseling: Through motivation, self-direction, self-knowledge, and relationships.* Thousand Oaks, CA: Corwin Press.

Stavros, J. M., & Torres, C. B. (2005). *Dynamic relationships: Unleashing the power of appreciative inquiry in daily living.* Chagrin Falls, OH: Taos Institute Publications.

Stephens, D. L., & Lindsey, R. B. (2011). *Culturally proficient collaboration: Use and misuse of school counselors.* Thousand Oaks, CA: Corwin Press.

Sterling, S. (2001). *Sustainable education: Re-visioning learning and change.* Bristol, UK: Green Books for the Schumacher Society.

Stone, C. B., & Dahir, C. A. (2004). *School counselor accountability: A MEASURE of student success.* Upper Saddle River, NJ: Pearson.

Stone, M. K. (2009). *Smart by nature: Schooling for sustainability.* Healdsburg, CA: Watershed Media.

Storms, B. A., & Gordon, A. (2005). Inquiry as a strategy for leading school improvement. *Educational Leadership and Administration: Teaching and Program Development.* (Vol 17, 59–74). CAPEA: Caddo Gap Press.

Strickland, D., & Riley-Ayers, S. (2007). *Literacy leadership in early childhood education: The essential guide.* New York, NY: Teachers College Press.

Stringer, E. T. (2014). *Action research* (4th ed.). Thousand Oaks, CA: Sage Publications.

Studer, J. R., & Diambra, J. F. (2010). *A guide to practicum and internship for school counselors-in-training.* New York: Routledge.

Sturken, M., & Cartwright, L. (2001). *Practices of looking: Introduction to visual culture*. New York: Oxford University Press.

Sullivan, A. (2010, November). Preventing disproportionality: A framework for culturally responsive assessment. *NASP Communique, 39*(3), 24–26.

Sykes, G. (1996). Reform of and as professional development. *Phi Delta Kappan, 77*(7), 464–469.

Taleb, N. N. (2007). *The black swan: The impact of the highly improbable*. London: Penguin Books.

Taub, J., & Pearrow, M. (2006). Resilience through violence prevention in schools. In S. Goldstein & R. Brooks (Eds.), *Handbook of resilience in children* (pp. 357–372). New York: Springer Science+Business Media.

Taylor, M. C. (1993). *Nots*. Chicago, IL: University of Chicago Press.

Taylor, M. C. (2007). *After God*. Chicago, IL: University of Chicago Press.

Taylor, M. C. (2012). *Refiguring the spiritual: Beuys, Barney, Turrell, Goldsworthy*. New York: Columbia University Press.

Taylor, M. C. (2014). *Speed limits: Where time went and why we have so little left*. New Haven, CT: Yale University Press.

Theoharis, G. (2009). *The school leaders our children deserve: Seven keys to equity, social justice, and school reform*. New York, NY: Teachers College Press.

Torbert, B. (2004). *Action inquiry: The secret of timely and transforming leadership*. San Francisco, CA: Berrett-Koehler Publishers.

Townsend, B.L. (2000). The disproportionate discipline of African American learners: Reducing school suspensions and expulsions. *Exceptional Children, 66,* 381–391.

Truebridge, S. (2014). *Resilience begins with beliefs: Building on student strengths for success in school*. New York, NY: Teachers College Press.

Ungar, M. (2004). *Nurturing hidden resilience in troubled youth*. Toronto: University of Toronto Press.

Ungar, M. (2005). *Handbook for working with children and youth: Pathways to resilience across cultures and contexts*. Thousand Oaks, CA: Sage Publications.

Ungar, M. (Ed.). (2012). *The social ecology of resilience: A handbook of theory and practice*. New York: Springer.

U.S. Department of Education. (2002). *Executive summary of the No Child Left Behind Act of 2001*. Retrieved from: www.ed.gov/nclb/overview/intro/execsumm. html

U.S. Department of Education. (2009). *Race to the top program executive summary*. Washington, DC: Author. Retrieved from: www2.ed.gov/programs/racetothe top/index.html

van der Veer, R., & Valsiner, J. (Eds.). (1994). *The Vygotsky reader*. Oxford, England: Blackwell.

Varela, F. J. (1992). *Ethical know-how: Action, wisdom, and cognition*. Stanford, CA: Stanford University Press.

Vavrus, F., & Cole, K., (2002). "I didn't do nothing": The discursive construction of school suspension. *The Urban Review, 34,* 87–111.

Vernez, G. (2008). Improving California's student data systems to address the dropout crisis. *California dropout research project report #10*, University of California Linguistic Minority Research Institute, University of California, Santa Barbara. Retrieved August 13, 2012 from: www.cdrp.ucsb.edu/pubs_ reports.htm

Voltaire. (1956). Candide. In H. M. Block (Ed.), *Voltaire, Candide and other writings* (pp. 110–189). New York: Random House.

Vygotsky, L. (1978). *Mind in society.* Cambridge, MA: Harvard University Press.

Vygotsky, L. (1986). *Thought and language.* Cambridge, MA: MIT Press.

Wakimoto, D. K., & Lewis, R. E. (2014). Graduate student perceptions of eportfolios: Uses for reflection, development, and assessment. *Internet and Higher Education, 21,* 53–58.

Wallace, D. F. (2004). *Oblivion.* New York: Back Bay Books.

Watson, L. W. (2000). Working with schools to ease student transition to the community college. *New Directions for Community Colleges, 2000*(111), 53–58.

Wenger, E. (2006). *Communities of practice, a brief introduction.* Retrieved from: http://ewenger.com/theory/

Werner, E. E. (1989). Children of the garden island. *Scientific American, 260*(4), 106–111.

Werner, E. E. (1996). How children become resilient. Observations and cautions. *Resiliency in Action, 1*(1), 18–28.

Werner, E. E. (2006). What can we learn about resilience from large-scale longitudinal studies? In S. Goldstein & R. Brooks (Eds.), *Handbook of resilience in children* (pp. 91–106). New York: Springer Science+Business Media.

Werner, E. E., & Smith, R. S. (1977). *Kauai's children come of age.* Honolulu: University of Hawaii Press.

Werner, E. E., & Smith, R. S. (1982). *Vulnerable but invincible: A longitudinal study of resilient children and youth.* New York: McGraw Hill.

Werner, E. E., & Smith, R. S. (1992). *Overcoming the odds: High risk children from birth to adulthood.* Ithaca, NY: Cornell University Press.

Werner, E. E., & Smith, R. S. (2001). *Journeys from childhood to midlife: Risk, resilience, and recovery.* Ithaca, NY: Cornell University Press.

West, C. (1993). *Race matters.* Boston, MA: Beacon Books.

WestEd. (n.d.). Student "fishbowl" focus groups. *Resilience and youth development module. California healthy kids survey.* Oakland, CA: WestEd.

WestEd. (2010). Student well-being in California, 2006–08. Variations by race/ethnicity in grades 9 & 11. Statewide results of the California Healthy Kids Survey. Closing the Achievement Gap Report. San Francisco, CA: WestEd Health and Human Development Program for the California Department of Education.

West-Olatunji, C., Shure, L., Conwill, W., & Rivera, E. T. (2008). Rite of passage programs as effective tools for fostering resilience among low-income African American male adolescents. *Journal of Humanistic Counseling, Education, and Development, 47*(2), 131–143.

Wheatley, M. J. (2012). *So far from home: Lost and found in our brave new world.* San Francisco, CA: Berrett-Koehler Publishers.

Whiston, S. C. (1996). Accountability through action research: Research methods for practitioners. *Journal of Counseling & Development, 74,* 616–623.

Williams, B. (1985). *Ethics and the limits of philosophy.* Cambridge, MA: Harvard University Press.

Williams, D. R., & Brown, J. D. (2012). *Learning gardens and sustainability education: Bringing life to school and schools to life.* New York: Routledge.

Willoughby, G., & Samuels, N. (2009). *Brilliant: The Heathside story: Appreciative inquiry in whole school transformation.* Chichester, UK: Kingsham Press.

Wilson, S. (2008). *Research is ceremony: Indigenous research methods.* Black Point, Nova Scotia: Fernwood Publishing.

Winkelman, P. (2012). Collaborative inquiry for equity: Discipline and discomfort. *Planning and Changing: An Educational Leadership and Policy Journal, 43*(3/4), 280–294.

Winslade, J., & Monk, G. (2007). *Narrative counseling in schools: Powerful and brief* (2nd ed.). Thousand Oaks, CA: Corwin Press.

Winslade, J., & Williams, M. (2012). *Safe and peaceful schools: Addressing conflict and eliminating violence.* Thousand Oaks, CA: Corwin Press.

Wittgenstein, L. (1953). *Philosophical investigations.* Oxford: Blackwell.

Wootton, D. (2015). *The invention of science: A new history of the scientific revolution.* New York, NY: HarperCollins.

Wright, M. O., & Masten, A. S. (2006). Resilience processes in development. In S. Goldstein & R. Brooks (Eds.), *Handbook of resilience in children* (pp. 17–38). New York: Springer Science+Business Media.

Wulf, A. (2011). *Founding gardeners: The revolutionary generation, nature, and the shaping of the American nation.* New York: Vintage Books.

You, S., Furlong, M., Felix, E., & O'Malley, M. (2015). Validation of the social and emotional health survey for five sociocultural groups: Multigroup invariance and latent mean analyses. *Psychology in the Schools, 52* (1), 349–362.

Young, A., & Kaffenberger, C. (2009). *Making data work* (2nd ed.). Alexandria, VA: American School Counseling Association.

Index

Note: Page numbers followed by *f* and *t* refer to figures and tables respectively.

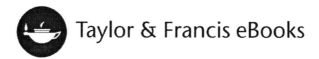